SUPER HEALING

SUPER HEALING

*Engaging Your Mind,
Body, and Spirit to
Create Optimal Health
and Well-Being*

Elaine R. Ferguson, MD

Health Communications, Inc.
Deerfield Beach, Florida

www.hcibooks.com

The publishers and author of this book make no medical or psychological claims for its use. The author does not dispense medical advice or prescribe the use of any technique as a form of treatment for physical, psychological, or medical problems without the advice of a physician, either directly or indirectly. The intent of the author is only to offer information of a general nature to help you in your quest for emotional, psychological, and spiritual well-being. In the event you use any of the information in this book for yourself, which is your constitutional right, the author and the publisher assume no responsibility for your actions.

Library of Congress Cataloging-in-Publication Data

Ferguson, Elaine R.
    Superhealing : engaging your mind, body, and spirit to create optimal
      health and well-being / Elaine R. Ferguson, MD.
        pages cm
    Includes index.
    ISBN 978-0-7573-1752-1 (Paperback)
    ISBN 0-7573-1752-9 (Paperback)
    ISBN 978-0-7573-1753-8 (ePub)
    ISBN 0-7573-1753-7 (ePub)
    1. Health.   2. Medicine, Preventive.   3. Diet therapy.
      4. Mind and body therapies.   I. Title.
    RA776.F38 2013
    613—dc23

                                       2013022886

HCI, its logos, and marks are the trademarks of Health Communications, Inc.
Publisher: Health Communications, Inc.
3201 S.W. 15th Street
Deerfield Beach, FL 33442-8190

Cover design by Larissa Hise Henoch
Interior design and formatting by Dawn Von Strolley Grove

To all who seek to improve

their health and well-being,

may you discover the power

that resides within.

CONTENTS

PREFACE

Good health is more than a body that works.
It is feeling good about yourself, dealing effectively
with people and situations around you, and growing
spiritually toward a new sense of wholeness
and meaning in life.

—*Anonymous*

WELCOME TO *SUPERHEALING*. WELCOME TO THE MYSTERY AND magnificence of your own body. In this book, you'll learn about research breakthroughs from different scientific fields that you can utilize to enjoy optimal health and well-being. This book is designed to provide you with the vital health-promoting information, tools, and techniques you need to unleash the remarkable, inborn healing capacity that resides within you. Is your life vibrant and optimal? Has it been awhile since you've felt really great? Are you sluggish and tired, lacking the energy you need to get through the day? Do you typically schlep through life, carrying your body along, but suspect that you must do something soon to prevent the development of a serious illness?

While you may be physically healthy, if you have been under stress without resolution for an extended period, then despite your best efforts, you're at risk of developing chronic diseases.

Do you feel ready to improve your health but don't know the right steps to take? Even though you may not have a physical illness just yet, perhaps you've become aware that you don't quite have the vibrant health you desire and deserve. Maybe you are currently living with a serious chronic disease, perhaps even one your doctor says is terminal. Whatever the case may be, isn't right now, this precious moment, an appropriate time for you to step up and take charge of your well-being?

The beauty of the superhealing approach to wellness is that it really doesn't matter what your current state of health is when you begin the program. Everyone can heal. Depending on how far your health is from ideal, you can either dramatically improve it or subtly but meaningfully enhance it once you understand what actions you must take. Vibrant well-being is your birthright. The challenge is learning how to create it, because if you're like most people in our society, you were never taught how to be healthy.

Are you facing the inevitable precipice of old age but want to continue to feel young? Are you looking for complementary wellness techniques beyond your conventional medical care to empower you to feel great? Or do you want something more for yourself but just don't know how to define it? In addition to addressing your own concerns, do you also want to help your loved ones experience improved health? All these are valid reasons to learn about the superhealing approach. And if I play my part well as your guide by presenting the breakthrough research now available to us, you can rest assured that this book will leave you with practical solutions you can implement.

We have all met someone who was physically sound but emotionally unstable and spiritually deprived. Perhaps you've even felt this way yourself at times, especially when life has put you under pressure. I know there have been times that I have felt this way, but I would have to say that these moments are fewer and farther between now that I am aware of the possibility of superhealing. Even though you may currently be focusing on improving your physical health, you can still be unhealthy in meeting your emotional and spiritual needs. The approach to wellness you're going to learn about in *Superhealing* can help you to turn your situation around so that your mind, body, and spirit are brought into balance. The scientific studies presented here will show you that when we neglect our emotional and spiritual needs, it is to our own peril, because that neglect is detrimental not only to our emotional health but to our bodies as well.

MEET YOUR AMAZING BODY

I'd like to introduce you to your amazing body. Volumes of encyclopedias couldn't describe the many wondrous activities that are going on within you right now as you are reading my words on this page. When you mentally scan your body, you are unaware of the thousands of biochemical reactions taking place or the creation and repair of your cells and organs. Nor are you aware of the vigilant protection your immune system is providing you. At this very moment, it is destroying all the invading organisms and foreign particles that could potentially cause you significant harm, while keeping an eye out for any changes in your cells that might indicate the presence of cancer. Fortunately, you don't need to be aware; everything I've just described is happening automatically.

We take our bodies for granted in many ways. We expect them to do what we want when we want: to walk, touch, digest, move, think, and creatively express our thoughts. We don't sit around wondering why or how the body can do these things. But maybe it's time we should. I know you are familiar with your body and its functions, but please allow me to introduce you to it in the most unusual and highly detailed scientific way—a way that is rarely thought of outside biology class.

- Your lungs contain more than 300 million capillaries (microscopic blood vessels).

- Your bones are as strong as granite in supporting your weight. A matchbox-size piece of healthy bone can support nine tons of weight—four times more than man-made concrete can support.
- The acids in your stomach are strong enough to dissolve metals like zinc, yet the cells in your stomach lining reproduce so quickly that your digestive acids don't have time to dissolve them.
- Each of your kidneys contains at least a million individual filters. Every sixty seconds, these filters purify more than two pints of blood.

And this is just the tip of the iceberg. There are so many more remarkable facts to discover that only a huge library could contain them. Your body has an extraordinary capacity to repair many of its own organs and tissues when they're damaged by either trauma or disease. For example, when you cut your hand, your body immediately launches a complex response to repair the wound and ward off possible infections that could be caused by invading organisms.

Along with other processes involved in this response, your skin cells instantaneously begin to divide and grow to fill the wound and restore the integrity of your skin. The cells adjacent to the wound are automatically stimulated to multiply. The DNA in the nucleus of each skin cell is reproduced with the help of some of the most remarkable chemical processes known to exist.

As your cells begin to multiply, your blood supply is enhanced to adapt to the unique characteristics of your wound. Your blood provides the chemicals that are required to help the skin cells grow: vitamins, minerals, and amino acids (the building blocks of protein). Then, once your skin cells have filled in the formerly wounded area, the replication effort is turned off in the cells, one by one, so that the skin cells don't keep on replicating beyond what is needed—thus, they avoid causing the creation of a skin tumor. Your body's cells know exactly when to grow and exactly when to turn off, so that when all is said and done, you're left with a perfect, or nearly perfect, replacement for the skin you lost when you were wounded.

Because your body contains such powerful mechanisms of biochemistry and energetic transformation that promote self-healing on a molecular level, all the aforementioned types of processes are capable of happening without your conscious awareness or involvement. Your body's ability to heal itself is so very powerful; in fact, you couldn't stop yourself from healing that cut if you wanted to! You can interfere with the process and slow it down, but your body will automatically do everything within its innate power to repair your wounded tissue.

You can't stop any of your body's other automatic functions, either. This makes it even more interesting that, as contemporary research has shown, your conscious involvement can and will enhance, support, and promote your body's innate healing processes, leading to superhealing.

Superhealing phenomena are what we are going to explore in this book.

WHY ARE WE ONLY JUST NOW FINDING THIS OUT?

Our bodies are naturally designed to express optimal health and well-being, yet most of us simply haven't been taught to engage this natural healing capacity to the best of our abilities. This is partly due to cultural forces, such as an absence in the West of a tradition of mental, emotional, and spiritual practices like meditation. In addition, there is the considerable political influence of the pharmaceutical and insurance industries and the predominant focus of conventional medicine on the use of drugs, surgery, and technology. It is hard to break the bonds of medical tradition.

In a 2000 medical journal article, Dr. David Sobel wrote, "Mind/body medical interventions are often held to a higher standard of evidence than are traditional ones, and must justify themselves not only by improved health outcomes and quality of care, but also on the basis of cost alone. Both medical and mind/body health interventions should be judged by a similar set of criteria, and the beliefs and biases that delay the use of psychosocial interventions need to be challenged."[1]

An ounce of prevention truly is worth a pound of cure, for so many reasons. Since prevention spares us the pain and suffering associated with illness, which can be debilitating and impede our lives and happiness, the comparatively few dollars it costs to implement preventive measures are far more valuable than the thousands of dollars required to treat a disease. In my opinion, the field of medicine is off center, and the influences of the pharmaceutical and insurance industries keep us from having access to the information we need to make the best lifestyle choices for ourselves.

Part of the reason I wrote *Superhealing* is to give you access to this vital, life-giving information. This book might challenge your beliefs. You will discover that you don't have to get sick, that your genes aren't fixed, and that your family's medical history isn't your destiny. It is how you live that plays the most significant role in your health; far more important than your access to medical treatment.

As you may already know, people are sicker today than ever before. This is ironic and tragic, considering the breathtaking advances in diagnostic technology and medications in the last few decades. In the twenty-first century, we Americans are developing chronic diseases at alarming rates and at younger ages. Adult-onset diabetes, or type 2 diabetes, was formerly unheard of in people under forty-five, but now it is a common occurrence among teenagers and even children as young as ten.[2] More young children now have fatty deposits in their arteries similar to the condition of people decades older.[3] Poor nutrition is fueling an obesity pandemic, and the cancers of old age—breast, prostate, and colon—now regularly occur in men and women in their twenties.[4]

Furthermore, we are seeing alarming rates of adverse drug interactions, medical accidents, and harm caused by embracing a technological approach to health care that appears to have run amok.[5] Medical costs, which are the leading cause of bankruptcy in the United States, are skyrocketing, and no relief is yet in sight.[6] It is therefore essential for you to take your health into your own hands.

Right now is the perfect time for you to learn some simple but powerful health-giving solutions that arouse your body's capacity for healing and regeneration. With our new comprehension of phytonutrients (plant nutrients), the biochemistry of emotion, and epigenetics (environmental and emotional effects on genes)—all evidence of the role of the mind and spirit in the health of the body—there is so much that you can do to create optimal health and well-being.

WHY I WROTE THIS BOOK

I've written *Superhealing* because I am committed to helping you learn how to correct imbalances while they are still relatively easily resolved, so you can maintain good health and prevent the development of unnecessary diseases. I also want to show you how to activate the healing response on every level of your being—mind, body, and spirit—so that they work together to reverse more advanced disease processes. As a physician, I feel privileged to have had the opportunity to witness the manifestation and expression on several occasions of the tremendous innate healing ability that everyone possesses. Its presence is awesome and powerful, and any description of it is merely a shadow of the experience itself. Nonetheless, it is real.

I've seen cancers deemed terminal suddenly disappear from bodies racked with pain and anguish. I've seen the dead return to life, their bodies remarkably unaffected by their death experiences. I've watched little children—premature babies too tiny to exist on their own outside an incubator—survive against insurmountable odds. These and other similar experiences have convinced me of the urgent need for the transformation of our philosophy of and approach to health and healing. These miracles of health and healing need to be available to as many people as possible—they need to be available to *you*—and they are, when superhealing is engaged.

During my first year in medical school, I was amazed by how the body works. I remember reading Arthur Guyton's *Textbook of Medical Physiology* and discovering the way that hormones are released and act throughout the entire body, like a symphony of intricate chemical molecules. While watching a movie on the functioning of the heart, I was awestruck. Can you imagine how powerful this relatively small muscle is to provide your entire body with the blood flow it needs to sustain life? It pumps an average of seventy beats per minute, 100,000 times a day, 35 million times a year, and 2.5 billion times in an average lifetime. Witnessing these profound displays of the life force made me wonder how the spirit interacts with the body. What intelligence is guiding it?

I went to medical school because I believed that I'd be taught how doctors help their patients to improve their health. Buzzer, please—

bzzzzzzz. That didn't happen, and I'm sure you can imagine that I was deeply disappointed. In my heart I knew that something very important was missing in my education. I never heard one lecture on how to create health during my seven years in medical school and residency training. Nutrition was treated like a passing thought. The glaring absence of health-promoting information in the curriculum was a painful reminder to me of the critical missing link. Medical school was all about managing the symptoms of disease.

Why isn't the training of doctors focused on health? That's a really good, complex question, and the answer can be summarized as follows: Business forces took hold of medical education more than a century ago, and since then the focus has been on pharmaceutical drugs, surgery, and technology. That's just how the allopathic (Western) medical system is set up. Conventional medicine has certainly made amazing strides in certain areas, especially in diagnosis, disease identification, drug development, and the treatment of acute diseases, such as infections and traumatic injuries. That's all important stuff. But I didn't learn what I knew in my heart I needed to know.

My strong desire to discover how I could help people—not only to reverse their symptoms but also to create true health and well-being—started me on a remarkable journey thirty years ago that has continued ever since. More and more of my colleagues have begun to take the same journey. A whole movement to integrate wellness practices into the medical repertoire and shift our emphasis to prevention is underway. Researchers have identified the significant roles that the mind and spirit play in sustaining our health and well-being, and others have validated the efficacy of relatively simple natural healing techniques. We now know that working on improving our health through the body alone is like sailing a sailboat with three masts with only one open. Healing becomes superhealing when all three sails are unfurled and catching the wind.

Throughout my three decades of practicing holistic medicine, I've often found myself in the position of answering the health questions of my family, colleagues, coworkers, and friends helped them to find simple solutions that remarkably improved their health and changed their lives, even though they were afraid to tell their doctors how they achieved the results. I have worked in hospitals and in private practice and have served as a public health advocate. My professional approach to medicine is holistic and integrative, and it includes a broad range of therapies that engage and empower my patients, from nutritional supplements and tai chi to volunteering, listening to music, and engaging in meditation and prayer.

I am a graduate of Brown University and Duke University School of Medicine, and I completed my residency training at the University of Chicago's Hospitals and Clinics.

I love to read, write, and express myself creatively in a variety of ways. But more important and meaningful to me than any of my achievements and credentials is my passion to help people live in good health and with tremendous well-being.

I believe your health is your greatest wealth, and your life, like the lives of others, is a precious gift. It is a blessing to be alive and to experience the joy that only thriving vitality can bring.

WHAT IS SUPERHEALING?

Superhealing is your innate ability to engage and accelerate your body's powerful natural health capacities through active participation in their expression. That means involving your mind, your body, and your spirit to restore the balance that is necessary to open the floodgates of healing that are not under your conscious control. This approach may require that you draw upon a broad range of clinically proven techniques, tools, and processes that speak to your needs and personal preferences. The superhealing approach affirms and recognizes that your essential nature is derived from your spirit, the foundation of all health and well-being.

A superhealing approach emphasizes the importance and necessity of involving the whole person, all aspects of being, in the creation of optimal wellness. Imagine a continuum of wellness, with optimal health and well-being on the far right and terminal illness on the far left. You can view superhealing as movement from wherever you begin—even a position of so-called neutrality, represented by a state of health that is seemingly okay but cannot be sustained—toward an increasingly positive state. This approach recognizes and promotes the fundamental innate capacity of the body to heal itself, and the role your various aspects of being play in the process. It acknowledges the role that all aspects of your being—your mind, your body, and your spirit—play in the expression of your health and the development of disease.

When we see superhealing occur in extreme cases, such as the spontaneous remission of a cancer, this innate capacity—perhaps more than any other mysterious inborn ability we possess—profoundly challenges the belief systems that most of us use to chart the courses of our lives. We can only aim to consciously create the conditions that make superhealing possible in any given case of severe chronic illness or injury; we cannot guarantee success. But the fact that healing is outside our conscious control and yet occurs can dissolve even our most carefully assembled belief systems.

As you read this book, you may realize that your own beliefs about what is and is not possible in terms of healing interfered with your progress in achieving optimal health and well-being in the past. I encourage you to use this reading experience as an opportunity to reach a new level of awareness, health, and well-being through a deeper understanding of your essential nature, which is the sustenance of life. *You are life.*

HOW TO USE THIS BOOK

Superhealing offers an in-depth look at the advances made by bold and daring medical researchers in recent years that confirm the power and efficacy of natural healing, a variety of approaches that sustain and uplift the mind, body, and spirit. I hope you will view this book as your companion, a friendly guide on your journey to optimal health and well-being. I have designed it to empower you with multiple options.

Part information, part inspiration, and part instruction, this book will allow you to create an individualized superhealing plan using a variety of clinically proven holistic and integrative techniques to reverse and prevent chronic diseases that are commonplace in our society: diabetes, hypertension (high blood pressure), heart disease, obesity, arthritis, acid reflux, cancer, and more. Its foundation is the thousands of studies that together demonstrate repeatedly the power of your body to heal itself. Even in the most dire and difficult situations, restoring your health is possible. You were born with this remarkable capacity. You are an amazing being, possessing the potential to overcome any illness. The superhealing approach intensifies and accelerates healing.

Health is not merely the absence of disease. It is a dynamic process, a harmonic symphony of biochemical, energetic, and psychological reactions occurring within your highly specialized anatomy as it interacts with your environment. Contrary to the prevailing scientific opinion, your body is not a biological machine. It can be likened to a garden or an ocean, an ecosystem whose elements must remain in balance if the whole system is to survive. Your mind-body-spirit needs balance and harmony, too.

The book has been organized into four parts. Part One, "Your Superhealing Mind," covers breakthroughs in science that reveal how intimately your mind is related to your physical health.

Part Two, "Your Superhealing Body," explores the latest research in nutrition, nature, and exercise, and it shows the influence your physical body has on your mind and your spirit.

Part Three, "Your Superhealing Spirit," reveals that the foundation of mental and physical well-being comes from a spiritual source. Although conventional thinking would lead you to view spirit and body as separate, every aspect of your spirit has an impact on your physical well-being.

Part Four, "Your Superhealing Lifestyle," will help you to develop a customized forty-day action plan to consciously engage your mind, body, and spirit and immediately activate your capacity for superhealing.

The path of superhealing supports the return of your conscious awareness of the harmonious state of being and the radiant light of your spirit within. In this place, disease, disharmony, distress, and pain are not known. The path of superhealing is actually an inseparable part of the life that is unique to you. There is no one recipe for how to journey along this path of awareness that leads to optimal health and well-being. Superhealing isn't only an outcome, such as the spontaneous remission of a disease. It is an alignment with an inner radiant healing force that speeds our movement along a continuum of health toward optimal well-being. The length of time required is truly not important. The fact that it happens is what matters, because once it does, it empowers and facilitates your progress toward the awareness of your true, primary wholeness.

Thank you for choosing to read this book and allowing me to share in your personal superhealing journey—your adventure. There really is no better time than now for you to discover the simple, powerful, health-giving solutions that *Superhealing* offers.

Welcome to the good health you desire and deserve.

ACKNOWLEDGMENTS

TO SIMPLY SAY THANK YOU TO THOSE WHO'VE ASSISTED ME IN THE creation of this book is a mere shadow of the heartfelt appreciation and gratitude I feel for all that I've received from those sweet souls surrounding me. First and foremost, I wish to thank the Divine Creator for inspiring me with the wonderful title and the uplifting and joyful energy that inspired and sustained me throughout this process.

I could not have done this without the love, encouragement, and unwavering support of my husband, Victor Johnson. I was catapulted by his faith in my ability, his respect for my passion, and his commitment to our family.

My parents, James and Lucile Ferguson, who dwell in my heart, provided me with the foundation to live a life filled with possibility and the expression of my dreams, including becoming a physician and healer.

To my sister, Denise: You are the brightest, shining example of superhealing in my life. Thank you!

I have the extraordinary blessing of a circle of friends that over the years has become a sphere of kinship: James Childs, Gina Israel, Joyce Nyongani, Ora Holmes, Annette Williams, Olga Padilla, Connie Harper, Bruce Butler, Rudy Lombard, Wendy Guess, James Gross, Robert Willis, Mitchell and Joyce Butler, Denise Slaughter, Sherry Faulkner, Brian Lacy, Rudy Lombard, Deborah Williamson, and Charles Collins.

I am also grateful to my two mentors, who came into my life during my adolescence: Darryl Pursiful and Levi Adams. They have remained dear wise counselors for several decades.

Finally, to Jill Kramer, my agent: You're a heaven-sent friend and advocate—thank you! To Angela Hynes and Stephanie Gunning: Thank you for being such wonderful midwives to this process and for sustaining me throughout the writing process. And to my editor, Tonya Woodworth: Your clarity and editing skills have made this book shine. Thank you from the bottom of my heart!

INTRODUCTION: The Foundation of Superhealing—the Unity of Mind, Body, and Spirit

The separation of psychology from the premises of biology is purely artificial because the human psyche lives in indissoluble union with the body.

—Carl Jung

IT WAS THE VERY FIRST TIME I'D EVER CONFRONTED A CANCER PATIENT. Just the thought of it made me nervous. Cancer is our worst, most ferocious enemy, the taker of life, the proverbial thief in the night, and the deliverer of unbelievable pain. I'd seen specimens of cancer in the lab and learned the details of how cells go astray, overgrowing and creating a path of such overwhelming consumption that the cancer leads to its own demise along with the body of its host. And here it was, finally, in the flesh.

I was on the psychiatric rotation, my first clinical second-year rotation in a hospital after the most intensive year of learning I'd ever known. My mind was filled with facts, figures, and theories that would be the foundation of my clinical experience as an eager medical student. On this particular day, I was assigned to interview a young woman whom I'll call Melissa (not her real name, of course). She looked healthy, but she lay in the bed listlessly. Unfortunately for Melissa, she had been diagnosed with malignant melanoma (skin cancer). In 1975, there wasn't much that medical treatment could do for her other than to attempt to postpone as long as possible the inevitable, painful death that lurked ahead.

1

Melissa was pretty, but her deep sadness, understandably, veiled her beauty. My assignment was to interview her to see whether there were any signs of a mental illness accompanying her terminal physical disease. She was sweet, cooperative, and probably very lonely, so my visit seemed to be a welcome relief from the glaring silence that otherwise filled her room. At age twenty-eight, Melissa was already the mother of four. She talked about her children and her husband much more than she did about herself. During those brief moments of expressing herself, she seemed to forget the death sentence that awaited her. Then reality returned, and she spoke passionately to me about her concerns about what was going to happen to her children after she died.

Listening to Melissa, I was speechless. Fear and regret streamed through me. I wanted to help. I wanted to grab her and hug her and tell her that everything was going to be all right, but I didn't because I knew I'd get in trouble if I did. As medical students, we were taught to be "distant" and "objective." What did that really mean? I thought it was cruel and heartless. But who was I to challenge the instructions of my professors?

As much as I wanted to help Melissa, I didn't know what to do or say to this suffering soul. I was totally inept at comforting her. I deeply wanted to relieve her pain, but I choked when I tried. The words just didn't come. I could sense her emptiness, her pain, and her way of making peace with her situation—if that's what it can be called to confront the inevitable. After our conversation, I rushed to find my supervising resident. "She seems depressed," I said to my advisor. "Can depression cause melanoma?"

"No," he replied emphatically, shaking his head as though insulted by my question. "There are only seven psychosomatic diseases. These are ulcers, hypertension, rheumatoid arthritis, hyperthyroidism, neurodermatitis, asthma, and ulcerative colitis."[1]

Well, I am not buying that theory, I thought, *at least not based on what I've just observed.* A kaleidoscope of other emotionally affected patients I'd met ran through my mind. *That's simply not true.* In my heart I knew better. I couldn't think of one patient I'd seen who wasn't emotionally distressed in some form or fashion, and it seemed a very good question to ask: Which had come first, the illness or the emotion? Could there perhaps be a dynamic interaction between the two?

Right then, at the very beginning of my career, I asked a question that would ultimately become a guiding light in my investigation of the superhealing phenomenon. Since then, I have read thousands of studies that support the idea of a dynamic interaction between illness and emotion.

MEDICAL RESEARCH HAS PROVEN THE PHENOMENON OF UNITY

Perhaps you are skeptical of the claim that the mind and the spirit can positively or adversely influence the body or that the body can influence the mind and the spirit. Well, I've got tons of evidence. Did you know that having fake brain surgery heals patients with Parkinson's disease just as well as real surgery does?[2] Or how about the following:

- More heart attacks occur on Monday morning than at any other time of the week.[3]
- Forgiving people you resent lowers your risk of having a second heart attack.[4]
- Blood sugar levels in diabetics can be reduced through meditation.[5]
- Optimists are healthier than pessimists.[6]
- Optimism and other uplifting emotional states can prevent the development of chronic diseases.[7]

- Helping a stranger improves your immune system and overall health.[8]
- The simple act of writing about an emotional issue can improve your health.[9]
- Group support can increase longevity among severely ill cancer patients.[10]
- Your mind can reverse the aging process.[11]
- Listening to soothing music can help your body to heal.[12]
- Tai chi and yoga lower the blood pressure.[13]

Each of these remarkable benefits was revealed by a recent medical study. All can be attributed to the body's phenomenal ability to heal itself through various biochemical pathways modulated by our thoughts, feelings, and emotions. As we begin to participate consciously in engaging these dimensions of our being, we begin superhealing, which begins to move us in the direction of optimal health.

WHAT IS OPTIMAL HEALTH AND WELL-BEING?

For centuries, being healthy meant surviving long enough to reproduce. During the twentieth century, the common conception of health evolved beyond the view that health is the absence of detectable signs of physical or psychological disease to include prevention as a goal. Today, our definition of wellness is becoming even broader and more encompassing. Society is beginning to see that optimal health really is a state of well-being and vitality wherein we are able to express our physical, emotional, intellectual, creative, and spiritual capacities as individuals in a manner that is harmonious with others, with Earth and all her creatures, and with all of life. Health is not an end point. It is a dynamic process involving the entire body; it enables us to fulfill our life purpose, to live fully and abundantly. It is a process that involves our bodies, our minds, and our spirits.

Health cannot be achieved through treating physical symptoms while ignoring the underlying psychological and emotional issues that are now understood to cause illness. To achieve a balanced state of health in an ongoing manner and develop an effective treatment plan for anything that ails you, you must be inclusive and take physical, emotional, and psychological factors into consideration.

Like wellness, disease is a dynamic process involving the entire body, even if only one organ system is seemingly affected. You don't have to be sick to be unhealthy. Because health includes your mental and spiritual well-being, you can be considered unhealthy if you are physically intact while emotionally imbalanced or devoid of a meaningful relationship with your spirit. Research has shown that hostility is a risk factor for heart disease and that loneliness contributes to the development of several diseases.

Becoming healthy again after an ailment or an injury depends in part on your willingness to accept responsibility for healing the disease or condition and to make a commitment to explore aspects of your experience that defy and interfere with personal wholeness. You must take care of your body, mind, and spirit.

Optimal health and well-being—the highest possible level of vitality and resilience and the strongest immunity—is not achieved by treating only the physical symptoms while ignoring the underlying psychological and emotional issues that cause illness. There is a crucial relationship among the physical, mental, emotional, and spiritual aspects of our being that each of us must embrace if we wish to significantly enhance our quality of life. Although the healthcare industry has failed, thus far, to cohesively shift the medical paradigm from treatment to effective prevention, there is no doubt that the latest research acknowledges that the vast majority of chronic diseases—including heart disease, cancer, diabetes, and high blood pressure—can be prevented.

Disease is the manifestation of an existing imbalance that an individual is unable to resolve on any level of being. It is caused and shaped by a number of influences that may or may not bear a direct causal relationship to one another. These influences have usually been present and adversely affecting the individual for some time. The creation of optimal health and well-being, as well as the management of illness, ultimately requires the individual to understand as many of these influences as possible.

WE HAVE FORGOTTEN WHAT WE ONCE KNEW ABOUT UNITY

Across the globe, since time immemorial, spiritual traditions have viewed the mind as a doorway to greater spiritual and emotional awareness and increased physical health and well-being. Mind, body, and spirit were recognized as integrated parts of our being for thousands of years, so healers employed mind-body techniques to augment treatments that promoted healing of the body. Ancient Greek physicians, for instance, used holistic and natural healing practices, including techniques that involved the mind, body, and spirit that were passed on to them by the Egyptians.[14]

More than 2,000 years ago, Hippocrates, the Greek physician who is considered the father of medicine, observed that certain personality traits were more common in people with cancer. Identifying these traits led him to devise a course of treatment.[15] As the first holistic physician, he considered health to be a state of internal and external harmony with the self and the environment. Many years ago, not long after my experience with Melissa, I was blessed to discover the concept of holism that Hippocrates promoted, which has enabled me to provide my patients with better care. I was surprised to discover that its ancient roots extended around the globe and were present in many cultures.

While mind-body techniques remained in use in the Far East, in places such as India and China, Western scientists threw the baby out with the bathwater a little more than 200 years ago. An unfounded belief in the separation of mind, body, and spirit became dominant in our culture because of a political desire for separation of church and state. The body was given to the scientists, the mind and soul to the priests.

The split happened in the mid-seventeenth century, when René Descartes—a lawyer, philosopher, mathematician, and scientist— proposed a theory of the innate distinction between mind and body that prompted a disregard of the more organic and holistic approaches of that time. It wasn't a purely scientific notion, but one that was created in response to an agreement that he had to make with the pope to get access to the bodies he needed to study by dissection.[16]

Descartes basically, and perhaps understandably, cut a deal with the Catholic Church that would allow him to continue with his studies and research. He publicly agreed that the body was separate from the mind and the soul. Those realms of our experience were relegated to the domain of the Church so that he could claim the physical realm as his own territory.[17] Alas, Descartes's bargain set the tone and direction of Western science over the next two centuries, which divided the human experience into two distinct and separate spheres of experience. This artificial perspective is the foundation of mainstream medical science as we know it today.

Because of Descartes's agreement, mainstream culture, including the vast majority of our physicians, remains largely ignorant about the important role that the mind and the emotions play in the development of disease and in the healing process. Therefore, for most contemporary physicians (like my supervisor during my psychiatric rotation), even the mere thought of considering the emotional components of disease while treating patients seems to threaten the scientific approach to medicine. Since the beginning of my medical education, I've known I didn't want to become that kind of doctor. Medical discoveries that do not involve drugs or surgery are often ignored or misunderstood by doctors, even when research supporting these discoveries is reported in prestigious medical journals.

In truth, the separation of mind, body, and spirit is not real, although we have long been led to believe that it is—and we have created our treatments accordingly. Remarkable discoveries are being made all the time now that prove there is so much more to what we are than we can see with our eyes. We don't even know yet what these discoveries mean, but I believe that in the future these will influence our treatments for all kinds of diseases and conditions.

Quantum physicists, beginning with John Stewart Bell in 1964, have done studies on the phenomenon of nonlocality. In *Healing Words,* a book that explores the power of prayer to heal (which several studies have supported), Dr. Larry Dossey explained, "If distant objects have once been in contact, a change thereafter in one causes an immediate change in the other—no matter how far apart they are, even if they are separated to opposite ends of the universe."[18] As he pointed out, we are currently discovering how this applies to issues of health and well-being. After all, our bodies, like everything else in existence, are made of particles. However, we can be assured that this phenomenon is not theoretical; it rests on experiments.

The evidence for Dossey's statement is fascinating. A 1993 study conducted by the U.S. Army Intelligence and Security Command determined that white blood cells removed from the body continue to have a persistent, invisible connection to those remaining in the body.[19] The army wanted to better understand the influence of emotions on systems that were far apart in location but remained connected.

Scientists scraped white blood cells from the mouths of volunteers. Then, using polygraph probes, they separately monitored the cells in their test tubes and in their donors. The donors were placed in a room and exposed to emotionally charged videos. While the donors were watching violent scenes, the polygraph probe detected that the donors' white blood cells in another room down the hallway also became extremely excited, despite the distance. The experiment was repeated with up to a fifty-mile distance between the donor and cells, and similar results occurred. This experiment gives credence to the belief that all things are connected through an invisible web of life—and things that were once proximate, as they are in the body, are even more entangled.

The army study, the studies of particles done by physicists, and Dossey's investigations of the power of prayer reveal a similar connectivity and all point to the same thing: at birth, each of us was given access to an infinite mind, a kind of intelligence that is greater than we are but of which we are a part. Although modern medicine would have us believe that the mind and the brain are one and the same thing, numerous valid studies have in fact clearly demonstrated that the mind is not limited to the brain or even to the body. Your mind is vaster than your body, and it is also nonlocal, which means that its effect extends far beyond your body and can be measured physically. In fact, your mind is a phenomenon related to the entire web of life.

Fortunately, a growing number of open-minded and occasionally surprised scientists are now causing a shift in our view of health and disease through their investigations. As news of their observations and findings percolate through our culture, they are quietly ushering in a dramatic paradigm shift by challenging the traditional view of health and disease and, in some cases, dramatically changing the assumptions from which we operate. We are witnessing changes of such epic proportions that I believe only hindsight will clearly show how earthshaking their significance is. Ours is a revolutionary era that's bringing the truth about healing into the open.

THE LIMITATIONS AND DANGERS
OF MODERN MEDICINE

In one of the most memorable lectures I ever heard in medical school, "A Tale of Two Cities," a guest lecturer on epidemiology (the study of disease trends) described a study by medical economist Victor Fuchs comparing health statistics from Nevada and Utah.[20] Although the study's participants from the two states were nearly identical in income level, education, and age, the states had strikingly different rates of disease and mortality. The healthier residents were from Utah. Fuchs determined that this could be directly linked to positive lifestyle patterns. The participants from Utah had good diets, exercised regularly, and avoided tobacco, excessive caffeine and alcohol, and drugs. Our lecturer concluded by saying that in the United States, the vast majority of chronic disorders—like heart disease, cancer, diabetes, hypertension, and stroke—can be considered lifestyle diseases. The government has estimated that 85–90 percent of these diseases are preventable.[21]

I was awed as well as confused by this lecture: awed because it showed we do possess the power to control disease, and confused because so little control was being exercised. I eventually developed the opinion that people don't modify their lifestyles to boost their health to optimum levels because they have excessive faith in the power of medications and surgery to save them from their own poor choices. They give up responsibility for their wellness to their doctors. As Donald B. Ardell asserted in *High-Level Wellness*, "The single greatest cause of unhealth in this nation is that most Americans neglect, and surrender to others, responsibility for their own health."[22]

John Knowles, the former president of Rockefeller University in New York City, suggested that people have been duped, either accidentally or on purpose. He wrote, "People have been led to believe that national health insurance, more doctors, and greater use of high-cost hospital-based technologies will impart health. Unfortunately, none of them will."[23] It never made sense to me why we would depend on medications, which have the risk of significant side effects, when other choices are available and more important. My confusion about our choices was reinforced by experiences I had in hospitals.

My first year on a ward as a real doctor, after graduating from medical school, was fraught with a constant mixture of chronic exhaustion, sleep deprivation, uncertainty, and fear. In the second month of my internship, during a typical on-call evening, something occurred that would change my thinking and my life forever.

As I was sitting at the nurses' station, around 8:00 pm, completing an admission of yet another patient, I noticed one of the nurses behind me in the pharmacy area preparing a bag containing a thick, ominous-looking brown fluid. Her crisp, white uniform glistened against the steel cabinets and countertops. A few moments earlier, she'd mentioned that she needed to prepare a child's chemotherapy. For some strange reason, she spoke out loud as she connected the brown bag of fluid to the intravenous (IV) line. "I need to be careful and not get any of this chemo on my uniform."

I was an intern, a newbie, fresh out of medical school and still wet behind my medical ears. Wondering why she'd made this statement, I asked, "Is that because you don't want to stain your uniform?"

"Honey," she replied, with a look of utter disdain, "are you kidding me? You think I'm worried about a stain? This chemo eats through cloth. I don't want to get any on my uniform because it will burn a hole in it."

And we're putting this in kids' bodies? I thought. *That's not right. There must be another way.* With that concern in my mind, in that very moment I knew I could not become the cancer specialist I had wanted to be up till then. That nurse's simple statement instantaneously eradicated every aspiration I had to become an oncologist, in the process permanently altering my professional career and direction.

In the midst of this deep disappointment—as I was wondering, *Isn't there a better way? Why do we have to give these babies chemicals that eat through cloth? Isn't there something that can help the body to heal?*—I also could hear my spirit whisper, *There is another way.* My journey to discover the power of superhealing began.

A few months later, still a medical intern, I'd been up all night in the intensive-care nursery caring for several very sick premature babies who had needed emergency deliveries. While on rounds with the attending physician, I was desperately trying to stay awake, or at least not fall asleep standing up (which I'd once thought was impossible but now knew was not). The attending doctor began an impromptu lecture on a research finding that the most significant factor related to infant mortality rates was not the availability of intensive-care nurseries to take care of premature babies but whether measures had been taken to improve maternal nutrition and health during pregnancy. Preventive strategies saved lives, and what we were doing was much less important.

I was flabbergasted. Exhaustion fueled my thoughts. *If this is for naught, then what am I doing? Why am I killing myself, taking care of these babies, working thirty-six hours straight every third night, only to discover that it doesn't lower the infant mortality rate?*

Now I understand the gift of that devastating information. It was another fertile seed planted in my mind of the desire to do more, which I would nurture over the years. As I did, it began leading me to find alternatives to the limited approach of our medical system. In the case of premature babies, for instance, scientists have discovered that putting the baby on the chest of the mother, skin to skin, and allowing them to bond, instead of putting the baby in an incubator, helps the baby to thrive. Premature babies who are exposed to the mother's heartbeat and warmth have breathing that is better regulated, have fewer infections, gain weight more rapidly, and are discharged earlier.[24]

Almost thirty years ago, the Government Accountability Office (then still called the General Accounting Office) estimated that 70 percent of the procedures used by doctors were ineffective. Coronary artery bypass surgery, for instance, has been used to treat heart disease (the leading cause of death in the United States) since the 1970s. A 1982 study conservatively estimated that at least one-seventh of all such surgeries could have actually been postponed or avoided altogether, which means that 25,000 operations per year back then were unnecessary.[25] Life was clearly prolonged by the procedure in only 11 percent of all cases. More recent research has determined that the vast majority of these surgeries, compared to other medical treatments, provided no benefit.[26]

It's my opinion that the situation hasn't changed since then. Today, in the United States, coronary artery bypass surgery is performed twice as often as it is in Canada and Australia and four times as often as it is in Western Europe, despite similar population profiles.[27] This means that American doctors are more apt to recommend this particular treatment, whereas their counterparts in other nations are less inclined to do so—and with good reason: Recent studies continue to find no significant difference in the outcomes from surgery and other medical treatments in the vast majority of patients with heart disease.

Lifestyle modification is a better way. Dean Ornish, a holistic physician and writer, demonstrated a highly effective approach to reversing coronary heart disease based on more than two decades of peer-reviewed research funded by the National Institutes of Health and several foundations. It consists of a major nutritional component to lower cholesterol, along with exercise, group support, and stress reduction.[28] Many studies of chronic diseases show similar long-term benefits for patients over surgery alone.

Several studies have highlighted the various dangers of modern medicine. These include the approval of unsafe drugs, the hazards of diagnostic technologies, the high incidence of unnecessary procedures, and the inhumane and frequently stressful way patients are treated. These dangers were compiled and reported in an article called "Death by Medicine."[29] Certain extreme treatments, such as chemotherapy or a stay in a hospital's intensive care unit, can actually cause post-traumatic stress disorder in those who undergo them.

What makes the situation so outrageous is that the healthcare industry has traditionally encouraged the American public to be passive consumers—to wait for developing technologies and new drugs rather than to accept the role they play in the expression of their own health and the origin of disease. The research clearly indicates that when consumers take responsibility for their health and actively participate in lifestyle modifications and decision making, they usually don't get as sick in the first place, and when they do get sick, they heal faster. Throughout this book, I will present evidence of this to you.

The truth is that modern medicine has made minimal progress with its purely physiological approach to healing, except in the treatment of infectious diseases and of acute and traumatic illnesses. In fact, many see that technology has played a significant role in disrupting the cornerstone of the practice of medicine: the doctor-patient relationship. There is an increasing awareness that our medical system—contrary to its mandate—is actually the leading cause of death and injury in the United States. Each year, 7.5 million unnecessary medical and surgical procedures are performed.[30] The number of people exposed to unnecessary hospitalization every year is 8.9 million.[31] The total number of iatrogenic deaths (those inadvertently caused by a physician, by surgery or other treatment, or by a diagnostic procedure) is calculated at close to 784,000 a year.[32] The number of people having adverse drug reactions to prescribed medicine while in the hospital is 2.2 million a year.[33] And this doesn't even consider the adverse reactions that take place outside hospitals, which aren't officially recorded.

In addition to the alarming rates of drug interactions, medical accidents, and harm caused by a technological approach to patients that appears to have run amuck—ironically and tragically, despite all of our culture's prescription-drug taking and technology—diseases are not being cured. In 2009, the annual heart disease death rate was 599,413, and the annual cancer death rate was 567,628.[34] In addition, because there are currently more than 78 million baby boomers in America, we have a large aging population and are therefore seeing an increase in dementia from Alzheimer's disease and other conditions.[35] Around two-thirds of seniors (age sixty-five and older) in the United States have at least one chronic disease and regularly see seven physicians.[36]

Our healthcare system is disease oriented and does not adequately treat chronic diseases because of its primary focus on the physical aspects of those diseases to the exclusion of all other considerations. With rare exceptions, doctors typically omit and ignore any consideration of the psychological, emotional, environmental, and spiritual factors at play in the development of disease.

Was it always this way, or did physicians simply change their minds?

REMEMBERING WHAT
ONCE WAS COMMON SENSE

Some of our predecessors understood the truth about the unity of mind, body, and spirit. In 1909, Sir William Osler, long considered the father of modern medicine, stated, "The care of tuberculosis depends more on what the patient has in his head than what he has in his chest."[37] It took almost eighty more years for other scientists to catch up with his groundbreaking observation. During the last fifty years, but in particular since the early 1980s, medical researchers across the globe have expanded the horizons of medical research by exploring healing vistas and theories beyond the current approach of modern medicine. The findings of thousands of groundbreaking studies now confirm what the ancient healers knew: Your body, mind, and spirit are one.

Since the last half of the twentieth century, scientists have been shattering the ideas that for centuries served as the foundation of Western science. In exploring how mind, spirit, and emotion are connected to the body, they learned that these aspects of our being form an intelligent integrated system that functions in a dynamic state of harmony. Our thoughts, feelings (defined as physical sensations), emotions (defined as physical sensations that arise with mental interpretation), beliefs, judgments, and expectations are physiological expressions of awareness and profoundly influence how we perceive, respond, and experience the world.

Recent scientific studies have made breakthroughs in understanding exactly how certain chemicals form a remarkable interactive bridge between the mind and the body. Pioneering research from a range of disciplines—including psychoneuroimmunology (study of the link between the mind, brain and immune system), psychophysiology, neurotheology (research on how religious practices affect the brain), epigenetics, and biology—has demonstrated how our responses to our experiences shape our internal chemistry by triggering and regulating neuropeptides (amino acid combinations that affect the nervous system) and their receptors.[38] These discoveries are revolutionary, and I believe they will be better understood and appreciated in the coming years. I will offer details about these studies in subsequent chapters so you can begin to understand their exciting implications in full.

By confirming the biochemical basis of emotions, these types of studies can empower you to unleash the incredible healing power of your thoughts. You can learn to recognize both how the mind expresses itself through the body and how the body expresses itself through the mind. When you respond to those expressions at the same time, you can initiate your superhealing capacity.

The truth is that the separation of mind, body, and spirit is an artificial, arbitrary designation.

THE ESSENCE OF THE SUPERHEALING APPROACH

Holism, wholeness, healing, and *holiness* are all derived from the same root in Old English: *haelen,* to "make whole." Superhealing is an integrative healing approach to transforming and transcending the physical, emotional, psychological, and spiritual limitations that have been imposed on us throughout our lives. These factors lead to imbalance and chronic disease if they're not addressed in a timely manner. Once we've transcended these limitations, we all have the inborn capacity to superheal our lives.

Because mind and body are inseparable, the vast majority of illnesses, if not all, carry significant psychosomatic components; that is, emotions have contributed to their development and progression. I believe that every disease has an underlying emotional, mental, or spiritual dimension that either directly or indirectly affects its course. Yet diseases don't have to be viewed in a negative, despairing light. Rather than being considered punishments, they can be considered friends, instructors, and blessings—precious gifts, even—because they can lead to discovery, unimaginable joy, and triumph.

In this book, my goal is to help you recognize that all elements of creation are inextricably linked to the greater whole, which is greater than the sum of its parts. The human spirit plays a role in guiding the forces and laws of the universe. One element of superhealing is a sacred regard for all life. Although it is uncommon for medical doctors such as myself to say so—perhaps from a fear of being perceived as nonscientific—superhealing is a by-product of reverence. This approach is founded in the view that love is the essential underlying nature of creation and ultimately the source of all healing.

Love is the essence of your spirit. It is the light that embellishes our being with life. Love is the most important force in the universe. It can lift us from disease, isolation, and rejection to superhealing, awareness, connection, and joy. Love is liberating and transformative. It has the power to release us from the chains that hold us captive to a life of inconsistency, fragmentation, despair, pain, and disease. Quite simply, there are no limitations to love.

We all need love, regardless of who we are or of our condition, position, or status. Love makes our world go around. As the sage Mahatma Mohandas Gandhi wrote, "Love is the most powerful force in the world, yet it is the humblest imaginable."[39] We are love. Love is the essence of mind, body, and spirit. Superhealing is a by-product of acknowledging the spiritual aspect of being, the divine essence of us, or the force of love, which manifests and guides our health and healing. It is love that fuels the body's capacity to heal and regenerate itself physically, emotionally, and spiritually.

You were created in the image and likeness of love. The essence of your being is a place where peace, joy, creativity, intelligence, and healing reside. At your essence, you are good, loving, and lovable, regardless of what you think or others may have told you.

In this book, I will interchangeably use the terms *spirit* and *soul* to indicate the core of your being that is a pure, loving intelligence. Your spirit is the foundation of your life. It is from this intelligence that the remarkable superhealing capacity you possess derives.

ARE YOU READY TO SUPERHEAL YOUR LIFE?

When I initially share with people the remarkable superhealing capacity they possess, many of the patients, workshop participants, and individuals I've coached have asked me a basic question: "How do I begin to heal myself? I don't know where to start."

I've heard this question from those in the throes of serious and sometimes life-threatening disease, from those in the midst of emotional despair, and from others seeking a fuller way of living. They attempt to leave behind stress-ridden lifestyles and unhealthy behaviors. They are seeking peace, healing, and new meaning in their lives from the terrain of despair within themselves. Many believe that a doctor, therapist, or healer can do for them what they cannot do for themselves. This is not true. Everyone, including you, has the capacity to heal whatever needs to be healed.

You are a superhealer. You have the capacity in this very moment—regardless of any other consideration—to engage your body, mind, and spirit and begin to improve your health and well-being in a most profound and dramatic way. It does not matter what has happened in your past, what your doctors have said, or what your family or friends think about your choices. What matters right now is that you've made the decision to superheal your life.

The notion of becoming responsible for your health may be causing you some confusion. Let me clarify. There's no need to blame yourself for anything that you're experiencing. If you're not experiencing your idea of optimal health and well-being, that has occurred in the absence of understanding the role your thoughts, feelings, and emotions truly play. Your disease happened in a vacuum, without your knowledge of its true causes. And even though you didn't choose to get sick, you can decide to get well.

The potential for superhealing is everywhere. It is a precious part of your birthright. It is the process of expressing the intrinsic wholeness of your spirit, allowing it to issue forth into your body and mind. The path of superhealing is not a course of extremes. It is one of awareness and harmony.

There's no magical formula that can or will release you from your responsibility or your suffering. You must authentically assess the areas of disharmony and disease in your life, for therein resides your power. Your honesty and self-awareness can ultimately lead you to optimal health and well-being. Although this course of healing may sound challenging, when you allow yourself the opportunity by removing your resistance, it is simple and the most powerful thing you can choose to do.

Superhealing fosters a heightened awareness of your perceptions of your emotions and brings an increasing clarity and evolving
awareness of the oneness and unity of life within yourself and all of
creation. The resolution of denial breaks down behaviors that have
prevented an honest assessment and transformation of old wounds,
and it soothes fears. It also allows you the great opportunity to heal
your fears and to confront painful memories that you've held on to
but that no longer serve your well-being.

This process fosters a growing awareness of honesty, forgiveness,
and completion. It is a process in which the newness of life and the
refreshing fragrance of love penetrates everything. This leads to
peace, contentment, and healing.

Superhealing emphasizes personal responsibility and active participation during the therapeutic experience. The ultimate goal is to
enable you to live life fully and abundantly. A superhealing approach
considers any disease to be an important message that you need to
deal with and explore with awareness, not as a victim but as a survivor
and thriver. Rather than focusing on the diseased portion of the body
or psyche, superhealing engages the broader aspects of life—including
nutrition, environment, intellect, emotion, lifestyle, and spirituality—
in the creation and maintenance of health and the process of healing.

Instead of the cure-oriented, symptom-suppression approach that
is the foundation of our healthcare system, superhealing is primarily
concerned with promoting health and well-being, preventing disease, and supporting the natural healing process. Because superhealing is a result of promoting healing from within, one therapy is not
recommended over another. It's holistic health and medicine on ste-
roids, because of its focus on empowering self-care through your active participation. Holistic medicine enables good health to emerge
and fosters autonomy. It takes into consideration you as a unique

and precious individual, not your body in isolation, and it addresses the cause rather than your symptoms.

All of the techniques and principles I discuss in this book arise from the underlying reality that ultimately your superhealing comes from within. It is a manifestation of your soul essence—the core of unconditional love.

***

SUPERHEALING WORK SHEET: LIFE INVENTORY

A key ingredient in the superhealing approach is paying attention to your inner life. Our world draws our attention to the outer reality. Consequently, we don't listen to or value the wisdom of our inner voices, which are informing us of what we are experiencing and what we need. With the following inventory, you can reverse that tendency.

To facilitate an understanding and awareness of your emotional needs, here's a quiz—one you can't fail. It's a series of questions about your life. There are no right or wrong answers, only honest or dishonest ones. Why don't you give it a try? Write down your answers in a notebook or in the space provided.

1. How often do you consciously engage your mind on a daily, weekly, or monthly basis?
2. How often do you engage your spirit on a daily, weekly, or monthly basis?
3. Why do you want to experience superhealing at present?
4. What is your idea of optimal health and well-being?
5. What is your vision of superhealing for your life?
6. Are you willing to make changes in order to superheal your life?

7. What unhealthy behaviors are you willing to transform?

8. What positive behaviors are you willing to enhance?

9. In general, are you content with your life?

10. If so, why? If not, why not?

11. What, if anything, would you change in your life at this time?

12. What are you passionate about?

13. What in your life makes you joyful?

14. Of those things, what gives you the greatest joy?

15. What causes you great regret?

16. What gives you peace?

17. What do you love?

18. Are you happy with your chosen vocation?

19. Are you happy with your friendships?

20. Are you happy with your relationship with your family?

21. Are you happy with your romantic relationship?

22. Are you happy with yourself?

23. What's more important to you, your opinion of yourself or what others think of you?

24. How would you characterize each of the following relationships?
    - Your parents
    - Your children
    - Your friends
    - Your significant other
    - Your coworkers
    - Your neighbors
    - The Divine, or God

25. Describe a significant memory you have of
    your childhood.
26. Name some of your best and worst qualities.
27. What would you do if you discovered that your
    life would end
    - In one day?
    - In one week?
    - In one month?
    - In one year?
    Describe the goals you had in your life, when you were:
    - An adolescent
    - A young adult
28. Describe the goals you have in your life today.
29. What area of your life would you really like to change?
30. What part of your life is difficult and challenging?
31. Why is that portion of your life difficult and challenging?
32. What are some important dreams in this life that you
    have yet to achieve?
33. If you could change your life, what would your new
    life look like?

Now that you've taken this quiz, you have a sense of where you are
and where you want to go. Throughout the book, we'll be exploring
how to put those intentions into action.

Part One

YOUR SUPERHEALING MIND

CHAPTER 1

YOUR SUPERHEALING
MIND-BODY CONNECTION

Remember to cure the patient as well as the disease.

—Alvan L. Barach, MD

THE HUMAN MIND IS CAPABLE OF ACCOMPLISHING SEEMINGLY IM-
possible feats. Have you ever seen its amazing superhealing power
yourself? You probably have, although you might not have thought
that what you were observing was illustrative of this phenomenon.
When I was a little girl, I was fascinated by photos of men from distant places resting on beds of nails. I wanted to know how they did
that, and I knew I was looking at something very special.

Years later, I was watching an episode of the television program
That's Incredible that featured an American yogi, and I had a similar response. He was sealed into a tiny Plexiglas cube and then dropped into
the deep end of a swimming pool, where he remained submerged for
almost half an hour. It was riveting to watch as the yogi emerged from
the box at the end of the time span unharmed and in good health.
How could he do this? He remarked that learning how to master his
breathing and alter his state of consciousness had made it possible for
him to control his body and accomplish his remarkable feat.

In 1979, Norman Cousins, the former editor of the *Saturday Review*,
published *Anatomy of an Illness*, one of the earliest books on mind-
body medicine. He had been diagnosed with ankylosing spondylitis, a
painful progressive degenerative disease of the collagen tissue—in his
case, in the spine—after returning from a business trip to the Soviet

Union in the late 1960s. His doctors identified heavy-metal poisoning as a possible cause of his illness. He recalled some research findings he'd read that negative emotions can cause biochemical changes that have deleterious effects on the body. As a result, he suspected that adrenal exhaustion from stress had lessened his body's ability to tolerate repeated exposure to toxic diesel exhaust fumes during his travels.

Based on the information in the study, Cousins theorized that positive emotions might create changes in the body that would enhance his recovery process, so he began a program to uplift his spirits through exposure to comedy films. When his continual laughter began to disturb other patients in the hospital, he checked himself into a hotel (with his doctor's approval) and hired a nurse to care for him. As an IV solution infused with large amounts of vitamin C flowed into his veins, he laughed for hours while watching films starring the Marx brothers and the Three Stooges. Cousins reported that watching these films decreased his pain and helped him to sleep better.

Significant changes in Cousins's blood chemistry were revealed. The sedimentation rate (an indicator of inflammation) was taken daily, both before and after his laughter sessions, and significant decreases were noted. With this combination of conventional and unconventional methods, he recovered. His controversial personal account was published in the *New England Journal of Medicine,* prompting an outpouring of disbelief and heated discussion within medical circles of the day. *Anatomy of an Illness,* which was an outgrowth of the article, became a bestseller.

Recently I saw a news story on television about a young woman in Maryland who lifted a BMW that had moments earlier collapsed on top of her father. Her remarkable physical strength, which arose only in the midst of the crisis and as a result of her fierce determination to help him, saved his life.

What did the yogi, Norman Cousins, and this woman have in common? Their minds were so intently focused on an objective that it affected their bodies' capabilities and helped them to adapt to stress. Other than being very committed and, in the case of the yogi, trained to focus, they weren't necessarily different from anyone else. During my years in medicine, I have on occasion witnessed equally special events: patients experiencing spontaneous healing from life-threatening illnesses. In such cases, I've noticed that most people who experience these types of remarkable outcomes possess an unflinching determination to get well.

I believe your mind is as powerful as the minds of these people, and I intend to show how your engaging it consciously is a fundamental component in ultimately enabling its superhealing abilities. You don't have to wait for a crisis to strike before you learn how to develop your mind. It is possible right here, right now.

One of the most significant keys to superhealing is transforming your unhealthy responses to stress into healthier ones, with the understanding that your amazing body is highly adaptable and has the ability to manage acute physical and/or psychological stress. Your mind has the remarkable ability to help your body heal and express optimal health and well-being, especially when you are consciously engaging it to that end.

WHAT IS THE MIND?

The mind is the complex of cognitive faculties that enable consciousness, including thinking, reasoning, perception, and judgment. Your mind is the seat of your conscious and unconscious awareness and the intermediary between your spirit and your body. It is the element of your being that enables you to be aware of the world and your experiences. It is your thinking-feeling component.

Many people, including most physicians, think that the brain is the center and source of the mind, or the faculty of consciousness. It is not. In actuality, the brain is a sort of relay station; it receives information from the environment through your senses and translates these perceptions into biochemical responses.

For the last few centuries, Western science has viewed the mind as separate from the body. This has allowed doctors to view the body as a machine and treat it as such. But the truth is that your body is a dynamic, living organism, which in many significant ways is created by the mind. Your thoughts and feelings alter your body's condition.

THE BIOLOGY OF STRESS

In order to actively engage your mind in superhealing, it is critical to understand the significant role stress plays in your health and well-being. Stress is a major factor in the development and progression of the vast majority of diseases, especially the chronic and severe ones afflicting millions of us, such as heart disease, diabetes, and cancer. Even so, the significance of stress is often overlooked and unappreciated by doctors and patients alike.

Your body has the remarkable ability to maintain balance and function without your conscious involvement. A portion of your central nervous system, the autonomic nervous system (ANS), is responsible for regulating bodily functions, like digestion, blood flow, breathing, and perspiration. The ANS is also called the involuntary nervous system, since you don't have to think about these functions for them to occur.

However, you can and do influence these functions through your thoughts, feelings, and emotions. Perhaps you've never considered how a frightening thought or emotion triggers the gurgling in your stomach, the accelerating and pounding of your heart, the tightening of your muscles, or the quickening of your breath. It's easy to take these things for granted and not pay attention to what it is actually signaling the need for such changes. Since they are spontaneous, it's easy to think they're not under your control.

Why can thoughts and feelings affect you so dramatically? Your body's remarkably intelligent design includes the fundamental ability to maintain balance.

During the early part of the twentieth century, Walter Cannon, a Harvard University physiologist, first proposed the now fully accepted notion that the body has a state of homeostasis: a self-maintaining, harmonious condition that responds to internal and environmental factors. Maintaining homeostatic balance is a key ingredient in maintaining health. Anything that disrupts the body's natural balance can be considered stressful. Fortunately, the mind-body system has regulators that enable it to adapt to stress.

The important point here is that your physical state is in constant flux, wavering about a homeostatic point that is your body's optimal condition for living. Disease results when factors, whether internal and/or external, persistently disrupt your homeostasis and it cannot adapt to them quickly and effectively enough.

Although Cannon was ahead of his time with this idea, he proposed that the personality was the controlling and regulatory aspect of the body. The subsequent work of psychoanalyst and physician Franz Alexander, who was interested in the psychosomatic nature of illnesses, supported Cannon's conclusion that many chronic illnesses are not caused by external factors but are due to continuous functional stress on the body. Both men's views contradicted the prevailing theory that bacteria, viruses, and external forces were the sole causes of disease.

Through research, endocrinologist Hans Selye, a Swiss scientist at

McGill University in Canada, made a significant discovery: he identified the physiological response to stress, which is regulated by the
brain with hormones. In 1956, he published a landmark book, *The
Stress of Life*, in which he noted that stress is an unavoidable aspect
of life, a response to the daily changes we experience, and the body's
reaction to any demands made on it. His discovery was termed the
fight-or-flight response.

Fight-or-flight is a state of protective arousal, an instinctive response to life-threatening situations. This happens when your perception of danger and experience of fear is triggered to release a cascade of hormones and chemicals that prepare your body to run from
danger or to stand your ground and fight. In stressful situations, heart
rate, blood pressure, and muscle tension, among other things, all increase. Most of us believe that the body's response to stress is automatic and that we therefore have no control over it, but in fact we do.

Whenever you experience stress, whether it is triggered by a physical, an emotional, or an environmental event, your brain attempts to
adapt the body to it by initiating a series of chemical reactions. This
response results in the release of stress hormones known as gluco-
corticoids and catecholamines, which stimulate your entire body in
order to protect you. At the core of this reaction is the hypothalamic-pituitary-adrenal axis, an interconnected network of endocrine
glands that regulates the production of the hormones that include
cortisol, adrenaline, and noradrenaline to name a few.

During the 1940s, another pioneering researcher, physiologist
Walter Hesse, studied a key structure in the brain, the hypothalamus.
He discovered that stimulating different portions of the hypothala-
mus produced two diametrically opposed physiological responses.
One area triggered the fight-or-flight response, whereas the other
created a state of deep relaxation, promoting physical restoration.

The second response is one of the body's protective, healing mechanisms. The body's changes during this relaxation response include the following:

- Slower heart rate
- Lower oxygen consumption
- Decreased muscle tension
- Lower blood pressure
- Brain wave changes, from beta (normal waking consciousness) to alpha (wakeful relaxation)

Relaxation on many levels can be stimulated with a variety of techniques, such as meditation, visualization, biofeedback, hypnosis, and controlled breathing. These ways are interchangeable if your ultimate goal is relaxation.

You probably have a good idea what causes stress in your own life; it could be anything from running late to having an argument to paying your bills. It is very difficult to clearly define stress, because it is a unique and subjective experience for everyone. But it has a negative effect on your mental and physical well-being. Any external stimulation that disrupts homeostasis can be identified as stress.

As early as the 1920s and 1930s, the term *stress* was used in some medical and psychological circles to refer to a mental strain, an unwelcome happening, or, more medically, a harmful environmental agent that could cause illness. Dr. Selye was the first to define stress as the "non-specific response of the body to any demand placed upon it."[1] He conceptualized the physiology of stress as having two components: first, the set of responses previously discussed, called the *general adaptation syndrome,* and second, the development of a pathological state resulting from ongoing and unrelieved stress.

Contemporary scientists, based on years of subsequent research, believe that the term *stress* "should be restricted to conditions where an environmental demand exceeds the natural regulatory capacity of an organism."[2] Despite the numerous definitions of stress, recovering balance and functionality is the key to staying healthy.

WHY YOUR BELIEFS AND PERCEPTIONS MATTER

William James, the father of American psychology, asserted, "The greatest weapon against stress is our ability to choose one thought over another."[3] He understood that stress is ultimately subjective, a fluid experience that depends on how we respond to the events in our lives, how we think and feel about whatever happens to us. But stress doesn't reside only inside our heads. The circulating hormones released into the bloodstream when we're feeling stressed dramatically affects every cell in our bodies. For this reason, stress is a leading cause of chronic disease, doctors' visits, and hospitalizations. Chronic stress weakens us and makes us much more susceptible to developing disease.

According to the American Academy of Family Practice, nearly two-thirds of doctor's office visits are motivated by stress-related issues.[4] The most popular prescriptions doctors write these days are for stress-related disorders. Millions of people regularly take anti-anxiety medication to ease the stress in their daily lives. Constant stress weakens the immune system's ability to ward off infection and destroy cancer cells.

The majority of Americans feel stressed on a daily, if not hourly, basis. As I've already pointed out, more heart attacks happen on Monday morning, between 8:00 AM and noon, than at any other time of the week. This clustering of heart attacks is uniquely human. Scientists therefore theorize that it is not linked to biorhythms, but due to the psychological meaning of Monday morning.[5] Monday morning is the most stressful morning of the week because it's when people return to jobs of minimal, if any, satisfaction and resume other pressures typical of working.

According to the American Psychological Association, workplace stress costs U.S. businesses an estimated $300 billion each year in healthcare costs and absenteeism. Studies have shown that stress causes 19 percent of employee absenteeism and 40 percent of employee turnover.[6]

Since 2000, annual surveys have reported increasing levels of stress in the general population because of the state of the economy, fears related to terrorist attacks, concerns about the environment, and other issues. Unfortunately, even people who are aware of feeling stressed don't necessarily know how to effectively manage it. Because there are so many concurrent sources of stress in their lives, they are finding it much harder to recover and return their bodies to a normal state of balance.

Whenever you're experiencing anxiety, fear, distress, depression, and frustration (as well as other challenging emotions, to a lesser degree), your thoughts trigger the release of the same stress hormones from your brain that would be triggered if your life were in immediate danger. This alters the physiology of every cell in your body. Any continued pattern of negative emotional responses to stress will contribute to prolonged physiological stress, which can turn into chronic adrenal stress and affect your health in devastating and measurable ways. It's linked to an elevation of inflammation markers in the blood and an increased thickening of the arteries, an indication of the progression of the hardening of the arteries known as atherosclerosis, which leads to heart attack and stroke. Prolonged stress can also elevate your risk of developing certain types of cancer and even dementia.

When we face long-term stress with an attitude of helplessness and pessimism, our constant negative thinking and emotions interfere with our bodies' natural restorative capacities. In the presence of these feelings of helplessness and despair, we actually create a helpless, hopeless body that is much more susceptible to disease. The release of excessive levels of stress hormones affects the immune system by depressing the production of antibodies and interfering with other physical functions. But if we face stress with a positive attitude, we enhance our natural restorative capacities.

Most interesting, is that there is such a thing as good stress. Stress is a response that helps the body to maintain its homeostatic balance in the face of perceived danger. On a short-term basis, this is helpful to us. Selye documented that stress differs from other physical responses by producing the same systemic changes whether we receive good news or bad news, whether the impulse is positive or negative. However, in an effort to distinguish the two, he called negative stress *distress* and positive stress *eustress*.

When we are stressed, we can move from an alarm state to a resistance state and to an exhaustion state, depending on our reservoirs of energy to cope with stress. Despite the frightening statistics, the truth remains that *chronic stress has no power over you*. The only power it has is the power you give it. If you respond in your own mind to the stressors in your life, approaching them with a positive perspective instead of a fearful, helpless, or guilty perspective, your physiology will dramatically improve.

Superhealing involves consciously deciding to express emotions in an honest way, instead of repressing them, and maintaining a positive and self-aware outlook. These are critical, potent factors in creating optimal health. Nothing can replace these decisions.

PERSONALITY, STRESS, AND
HEALTH: ADAPTABILITY TO LIFE

I'd been in private practice for a couple of years when one day, while running errands, I crossed paths with the granddaughter of one of my patients. This particular patient, an elderly woman, had numerous medical problems, including heart disease, diabetes, and high blood pressure. In response to my question of how her grandmother was doing, the young woman quickly replied, "Grandma's fine. She only gets sick when she gets upset." That astute and timely observation struck me as a tremendous revelation. It made me consider my other patients in a new light of understanding.

When we are ill, how we respond to the illness greatly affects how well we feel. Hippocrates said, "I would rather know the person who has the disease than know the disease the person has." Studies have found that personality traits have an effect on long-term cancer survival. In a study to predict survival rates in terms of remission, the researchers found that personality classification could predict medical outcomes in 88 percent of the patients who had a rapidly progressing cancer. The most important characteristic was the "inability to relieve anxiety or depression." Only 46 percent of people with a poor ability to cope went into remission. Of those with a "fighting spirit," 75 percent experienced a positive outcome.

At the turn of the twentieth century, William James wrote, "The greatest discovery of my generation is that human beings can alter their lives by altering their attitudes of mind."[7] Since then, numerous studies have found that personality patterns appear to play a role in the regulation of the immune system and have shown that they can lead to the development of specific diseases. I discovered an interesting study from as long ago as 1937 that evaluated the coping styles that lead to disease. In this study, Harvard researchers found that individuals who typically handled stress and strain in an "immature way" became ill four times more often than those who didn't. Their chief coping style, projection—unconsciously disavowing their conflicting thoughts and feelings by identifying them in the behavior or statements of others—was like that of children.[8]

From 1947 to 1964, Caroline Bedell-Thomas and Karen Rose conducted a study of essential hypertension and coronary artery disease, charting its occurrence among 1,300 students at Johns Hopkins School of Medicine.[9] The researchers were most intrigued by what the study revealed about the link between personality and illness. The subjects of the study who had been emotionally distant from one or both of their parents for more than thirty years had unusually high rates of mental illness, suicide, and death from cancer.

Part of Bedell-Thomas and Duszynski's study consisted of giving students the famed Rorschach inkblot personality test. Students who developed hypertension, who had heart attacks, and who developed malignant cancers at a much higher rate had described the inkblots using "morbid" words. Those who later committed suicide had used cancer-related descriptive words fourteen times more often than their healthy counterparts had.[10]

Bedell-Thomas and Duszynski wondered, "Could unconscious dreads and morbid fears, which, in some individuals, are ever-present stresses, undermine the biological guardians of general resistance?"[11]

During my own medical school education, there was a lot of buzz about the type A personality. This personality style describes people who are obsessed with time management and are high-achieving workaholics, rigidly organized, and status-conscious. The three major emotional symptoms of this personality type are free-floating hostility, triggered by even insignificant events; impatience from a heightened sense of time urgency; and a highly competitive drive, which causes stress.

At the time my colleagues and I were buzzing about the type A personality, it was believed to be a significant risk factor for the development of heart disease. A long-term study by cardiologists of men ages thirty-five to thirty-nine estimated that the risk of coronary heart disease was doubled in those with type A behavior patterns.[12] For the first time in my medical education, I learned that personality could influence disease.

Years later, I would discover that the only real disease-predicting aspect of type A personality is hostility. Follow-up research determined that anger, hostility, aggression, a generally resistant and stubborn attitude, and defiance of authority have been found to be positive predictors for developing disease. Other traits of the type A personality may be related to heart disease but are not shown to directly cause it.[13] "The consensus is really that it is not all aspects of type-A behavior, but just the hostility component" that causes coronary heart disease, said Redford Williams, the director of the behavioral medicine research center at Duke University School of Medicine.[14]

Researchers have determined that hostility, independent of its contribution to unhealthy behaviors, contributes to the development of heart disease through increased blood pressure, erratic heart rate, fat accumulation, and abnormal platelet function—which means that it plays a role in the clot development that causes a heart attack.[15] Studies reveal that besides hostility, anxiety, depression, and low levels of social support also may be risk factors in the development of cardiovascular disease.[16]

It is true that we still do not know exactly what role the mind plays in maintaining strong immunity and preventing the progression of most diseases. However, considerable evidence has shown that the mind matters when fighting cancer. Research by many scientists is contributing to a growing body of information about the dynamics of the psychological, emotional, and social factors that affect the progression of cancer.

A recognition of the link between the emotions and cancer dates back to ancient civilizations. Hippocrates, whose approach focused on holistic methods and incorporating the healing power of nature, encouraged his fellow physicians to support and not interfere with the body's ability to heal itself. Around 170 CE, the prominent Roman physician Galen said that melancholic (sad) women suffer from cancer more frequently than sanguine (cheerful) women do. Although many of Galen's conclusions have been proven false over time, his sense of a connection between personality and cancer was astute.

In 1926, psychologist Elida Evans published *A Psychological Study of Cancer*, a book based on research into the link between depression and cancer. She advised that cancer is a signpost in the road of life calling for change.[17] During the 1960s, psychologist Lawrence LeShan conducted interviews with hundreds of cancer patients and found commonalties among them, including emotional repression, low self-esteem, long-term suffering, and the experience of personal loss.[18]

During clinical rotations in the hospital, I often heard my attending residents remark, "Only the nicest people get cancer." My observations confirmed what they said. Cancer patients, more than others, are usually extremely agreeable, pleasant, and solicitous. Why? Is there such a thing as a cancer personality, a type C?

Psychologist Lydia Temoshok did a study of cancer patients to explore the mind-body connection. When her results were released in 1987, she was accused of "blaming the victim" because she found a correlation between cancer and an extremely emotionally repressed coping style that involves appeasing others, denying one's own feelings, and conforming to social standards.[19] Type C patients were devoted to pleasing their spouses, clients, siblings, friends, and coworkers. Their core identities seemed to hinge upon gaining the acceptance of the significant individuals in their lives. This coping style seems to weaken the immune system's defenses and can render a person more vulnerable to cancer progression.[20]

What Dr. Temoshok was pointing to was a characteristic known as *other-directedness*. Sociologist David Riesman coined this expression in his 1950 book *The Lonely Crowd* to describe the psychological effect of always adapting oneself to another person. People who are extremely other-directed are out of touch with their own emotions and needs and typically look outside themselves for acknowledgment and direction. Unfortunately for them, physical health can be compromised by routinely repressing their important needs. As Dr. Temoshok noted, this type of person "is not aware that he or she is in distress while focusing on others. Since this pattern develops in childhood as a means of survival, during adulthood this pattern can make some social relations easier, but at a cost to the individual."[21]

Seeing how hard it was for people to change this pattern of behavior, Dr. Temoshok developed a program called Type C Transformation for cancer patients and for healthy people who want to prevent disease. Her program involves "gradual, stepwise alterations in the person's automatic responses, which facilitate transformation on cognitive, behavioral, and emotional levels."[22]

The emotional responses that are believed to predispose a person to the progression of cancer are prolonged depression, impaired emotional outlets, and rejection or abandonment by a parent or another significant person. Patterns of excessive denial, avoidance, repression, defensiveness, and rigidity of thought are associated with compromised immunity. This does not mean that emotional repression will cause cancer in every case, only that this behavior pattern is a risk factor for cancer and impedes the chances of recovery.

The three basic elements of transformation that type C patients benefit from are social support, personal empowerment, and emotional expression. Dr. Temoshok found that patients who underwent transformation surpassed their doctors' expectations for physical recovery.[23]

CONTROL AND HARDINESS STUDIES

When exposure to stress is prolonged, or when several sources of stress exist concurrently, it's hard for the body to return to a normal, healthy state of balance. Animal studies, as unkind as they are, have borne this out. In one, animals were implanted with tumors and then repeatedly shocked with electricity, a highly stressful event. If the animals could end the shocks, they were more often able to reject their tumors.

How does this translate into the stress of ordinary daily life for human beings? Ellen Langer, a Harvard research psychologist, determined that residents in a nursing home who felt no control over their daily lives, in terms of choices, experienced a much higher rate of death during the study than those who made choices. When the residents in her study were allowed to choose their meals and when they made telephone calls, their rate of dying dropped a full 50 percent within eighteen months.[24]

In the 1970s, Salvatore R. Maddi, a University of Chicago professor of psychology, read an article in the popular consumer magazine *Family Circle* that warned, "Stress can kill you, so you need to stay away from it." He wasn't certain of this assertion, because he'd previously conducted research that determined that stress could sometimes have a positive effect by stimulating creativity in those who didn't seek to avoid change. His research—different studies conducted in the last thirty years—has proven that stress can be beneficial when it's treated as a challenge. People who handle stress well share key personality traits, which Dr. Maddi calls "hardiness attitudes and skills."[25]

From 1975 to 1987, Maddi conducted a landmark study of mid-level executives at Illinois Bell Telephone, a division of AT&T. In 1981, they faced losing their jobs as a result of the breakup of AT&T. Because it was an extremely stressful time for so many executives, the number of heart attacks skyrocketed, to the point that a coronary care unit was created at Illinois Bell's corporate headquarters. Two-thirds of the managers fell apart from the stress of the company's downsizing. They had heart attacks and strokes, suffered depression and anxiety, and got divorced. But within this group of executives, there were also those who thrived in the face of severe adversity.[26]

Although the managers in the second group were similar in age and ethnicity to their counterparts, they held a different perspective. Among the managers experiencing high levels of stress, those who showed "hardy attitudes" experienced fewer mental and physical illness symptoms. Those attitudes entailed a commitment to the job, an amazing sense of challenge, excitement in response to adversity, and a critical perception of self-control. These managers didn't just survive, they thrived! They also rose to the top at Illinois Bell or at competing companies.[27]

The point is that no matter how bad things get, if you're committed, you will stay involved and give your best effort rather than pulling back. If you are strong in the attitude of control, you will tend to perceive yourself as in charge of your destiny, and you will try to influence the outcome of events rather than lapse into passivity. You thereby have the greatest likelihood of influencing the outcomes occurring around you. Sinking into passivity and powerlessness seems pointless to those with hardiness traits.

If you believe that change is normal, you will be more able to treat change simply as a challenge. If you are strong in the attitude of challenge, you will think that your life will be most fulfilled if you continue to learn and grow in wisdom from your experiences, whether they are positive or negative.

Together, the attitudes of commitment, control, and challenge provide the foundation for turning stress from an emotional disaster into a growth opportunity. Dr. Maddi believed that the hardy attitudes of commitment, control, and challenge are the best descriptions of human courage in action.[28]

Several additional studies have demonstrated that hardiness moderates the stress-disease relationship. In combination with social support and physical exercise, hardy attitudes provide protection from stress-related illnesses, despite genetically inherited vulnerabilities to certain diseases. Research psychologist Paul Bartone was commissioned by the U.S. Army to study military personnel in various stressful circumstances, including peacekeeping and combat missions. He found considerable evidence that the less hardy the attitudes were, the greater the likelihood was that life-threatening stresses and the culture shock of military engagement abroad would lead to mental breakdowns such as depression and post-traumatic stress disorder.[29]

From all these studies, we can conclude that our behavior, guided by our personality traits, influences the way we live and how well we can adapt to life's unpredictable trials and tribulations. Our perceptions, attitudes, and emotions are the keys to open either the doorway to health or the doorway to disease.

But how do we open the doorway to health? In the next chapter, we'll look at some recent scientific breakthroughs that show how to activate the superhealing mind-body connection that leads to optimal well-being.

SUPERHEALING WORK SHEET:
ASSESSING YOUR STRESS

For the next week, monitor your stress level and your thoughts, feelings, and emotions. Reflect upon the following questions or write about them in a journal:

1. How often do you feel stressed on a daily basis?
2. How often do you feel stressed during a week?
3. Describe a typical stressful situation.
4. What are the causes of your stress?
5. Of these causes, which are the most significant?
6. Is your stress increasing?
7. What are the signs and symptoms of the stress that you experience?
8. What physical symptoms do you experience?
9. What do you do when you're aware of your stress?
10. Do you think you ever experience stress but are not aware of it?
11. How do you engage your body, mind, and spirit when you're stressed?
12. Do you think your stress is determined by forces beyond your control, or does the way you view experiences determine your body's response to events?
13. Does stress create a sense in you of having a challenge to overcome or a feeling of being overwhelmed?
14. In your experience, are all stressful experiences harmful? If yes, explain why, and if no, explain why not.
15. What are some of the benefits of your stress?
16. If you were to respond in a healthier way to a particular stressful situation, imagine and describe how that response would feel.

CHAPTER 2

SUPERHEALING MIND-BODY RESEARCH BREAKTHROUGHS

The real voyage of discovery consists not in seeking new lands but in seeing with new eyes.

—Marcel Proust

FOR THE VAST MAJORITY OF HIS LIFE, JAMES WAS THE PICTURE OF health and well-being. At eighty-four, he was still very much the strong tower of the man he had always been. He looked like he was in his midsixties and was much fitter than men who were decades younger. He was full of life, with minimal aches and pains, thanks to his zest for life and his pursuit of hobbies and education. He had taken vitamins since his midfifties and engaged in vigorous activity, including running a landscaping business and maintaining a large organic garden that provided him and his neighbors with pounds of healthy fruits and vegetables. He had returned to his hometown in South Carolina to farm on the land he loved three years earlier, and he lived alone. He was self-sufficient and happy.

In his entire life, James had spent only one night in the hospital. He did all the right things. He gave of himself to friends, family, and anyone else who needed a helping hand. Yet a few days after being kidnapped and robbed of $10,000, he quickly deteriorated mentally and emotionally, because he was traumatized by the experience.

Nothing eased James's distress. He had lost his center, his sense of safety. The kidnappers had robbed him not only of his money but also of his enduring faith and trust in people. From the sidelines, I watched helplessly as he was diminished by the severe stress of remembering, every day, the painful incident he'd endured. A few weeks later, James had a panic attack and died from a massive heart attack.

He was my dad. I believe he died because he was overwhelmed by the distress caused by his terrible experience.

Distress is the silent epidemic of our time. The human body—which is exquisitely sensitive to the barometer of our thoughts, emotions, and especially our perceptions (our subjective interpretations)—is always expressing a dynamic symphony of responses. These are not limited to one part or portion of the body but are a global experience. Our thoughts and feelings initiate the electrochemical reactions that regulate our bodies' functions and set the tone for our quality of life. Anything that disrupts our minds also disrupts our emotions and our bodies. If we continually fail to adapt to any given disruption, whether it comes from inside us or outside us, we will experience chronic distress and potentially develop a disease.

The problem of stress is like a two-ton elephant sitting in the middle of the healthcare living room. It remains inadequately addressed by the medical community. Beyond interventions with antianxiety medication and the establishment of worksite fitness and relaxation programs, stress-reduction efforts have been marginal in our culture. The public health implications are so grave that we continue to ignore stress at our own peril. Stress is a reality that is not going away; there is simply more stress today than ever, coming at us from every direction in our world.

Trust me—you can't afford to ignore the sources of stress in your life. No one else can take on this challenge for you. It is your personal responsibility to learn to manage your own stress in a healthy way. No drug could ever do for you what your own calm and peaceful mind can do.

What are you thinking about? What do you feel? Do you pay attention and respond appropriately to your thoughts and emotions? What is the nature of your self-talk: Is it critical or supportive? Though seemingly simple questions, these are the keys to shifting your mind, and thus your body, to a higher state of functioning. How you think and feel from moment to moment is always being reflected in your physiology. To engage your superhealing mind, it is critical to uplift your thoughts to positive ones.

My hope is that understanding how your cells respond to your thoughts will empower you to transform your health for the better. The breakthroughs in mind-body research that we'll explore in this chapter are so promising because they show how the mind operates as a kind of interface between the body and the spirit. Like a rainbow bent back upon itself, with the many colors representing different facets of personal experience, the mind-body-spirit system is a dynamic, two-way communication loop. Body and spirit are continuously "talking" to each other through the pathways of the mind.

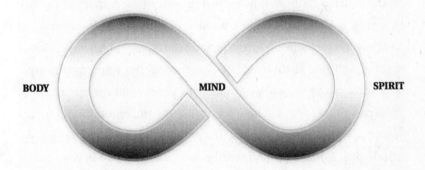

BODY   MIND   SPIRIT

Your spirit is the intangible core of your being. Everything you experience comes from your spirit. It is the point of origin that both establishes and guides your body and mind to be as they are; it is a blueprint through which energetic information expresses itself. It establishes communication with the body through the mind's inter-pretation and receiving shifting of spiritual qualities like love, peace, and joy. You experience these qualities emotionally when your mind-body-spirit system is in balance.

Your body communicates with your spirit about your environment through your perceptions. Everything you perceive with your senses is interpreted by the filter of your awareness and assessments—your cognition. Some of this mental activity is conscious, and some is unconscious. But no matter what you focus on by choice or by habit, your brain establishes pathways of neural activity to support and sustain your focus.

The emotions you feel are not just sensations; they are an entire set of electrical, chemical, and hormonal responses that are uniquely and identifiably your own. You create them based on how you build your brain pathways throughout your life. Emotions are the result of your interpretations of what you sense and what you believe. A lot of people—including me, years ago—have difficulty accepting that their thoughts have such a powerful effect on their bodies. But the reality is that a thought is never just in your head. A thought always triggers a cascade of matching physiological responses mediated by a variety of mechanisms. These include the release of neuropeptides, short amino acid chains that circulate throughout your entire body.

Although your body also influences your mind, in this chapter we're just going to look at how your thoughts and emotions influence your body on its deepest levels. The natural condition of your body-mind-spirit is harmony and well-being. As you engage in new, more beneficial ways of thinking and learn to alter your beliefs and subdue the stress response, you will begin to create an emotional style, personality traits, habits, and behaviors that will buffer you against the perils of chronic or severe stress. Engaging your mind in these ways will put you on the road to superhealing.

The good news is that you can develop enough conscious control to restore or sustain the natural harmony of your mind and your emotions, and balancing thoughts and emotions can improve your physiological health. Optimal wellness is associated with high mental performance, low stress, emotional stability, resilience, strong immunity, and a sense of vitality. If you manage your stress in a positive way, using mind-body interventions, you will have laid the foundation for superhealing in your life. Nothing can supplant this effort—not exercise, not diet, not taking supplements.

THE MOLECULES AND ENERGETICS OF EMOTIONS

Your emotions are mediated in part by a portion of your brain known as the limbic system. The hypothalamus, which is the endocrine system's master gland, reads chemical messages that can have certain effects on the immune system. For example, if chronic stress produces an emotional response of sorrow and hopelessness, it can suppress the immune system's ability to function. We know this because in pioneering research done in the 1980s, neuropharmacologist Candace Pert, a brain researcher at Georgetown University Medical School, discovered what she called the "molecules of emotions," neuropeptides. These chains of amino acids, located within the central nervous system and throughout the body, regulate key physiological responses that affect our ability to heal or develop disease.[1]

Dr. Pert described the manner in which our emotions are translated into chemistry and how the brain's opiate receptors, which are the cellular binding sites for endorphins (neurochemicals that have been called "nature's painkillers"), have a vital connection to human well-being. Therefore, she postulates that emotions are the links between mind and body that influence health. It is through the emotions we feel as a result of our thoughts and attitudes—or more precisely, the neurochemical and bioelectrical changes that accompany these emotions—that our minds acquire the power to influence whether we get sick or remain well. She wrote, "The same chemicals that control mood in the brain control the tissue integrity of the body."[2]

Pert's theory rests on the fact that neuropeptides are found throughout the body, including in the brain and the immune system. They are the means by which all cells in the body communicate with one another. This communication includes brain-to-brain messages, brain-to-body messages, body-to-body messages, and body-to-brain messages. Individual cells, including brain cells, immune cells, and other body cells, have receptor sites that receive neuropeptides. The kinds of neuropeptides available to cells are constantly changing, reflecting variations in our emotions.[3]

Pert wrote, "Neuropeptides and their receptors thus join the brain, gland, and immune system in a network of communication between brain and body, probably representing the biochemical substrate of emotion. Cell receptors are the interface between our emotions and our cells."[4]

THE NEW SCIENCE OF EPIGENETICS

Our genes were once thought to be the predetermining factor of our health, but now it appears that even these may be altered by the chemistry of our positive and negative emotions. From the work of molecular cellular biologists, we now know that our DNA is controlled by energetic messages received from sources external to the cells.[5]

In the last few years, the field of epigenetics has dramatically changed the way we view DNA, the underlying structure of our genes. The Greek-derived prefix *epi*—means "over" or "above." Consequently, the literal meaning of epigenetic control is "control above the genes." The study of epigenetics reveals that we are not the victims of our genes but rather their masters.

Since 1953, when James Watson and Francis Crick (and the usually unacknowledged Rosalind Franklin) discovered DNA, the building blocks of our genes, we've been led to believe, without proof, that our DNA is fixed. Furthermore, we've been told that it controls the traits passed to us by our parents, including our likelihood of developing a variety of chronic diseases. As recipients of genetic predeterminations, we've been taught, we are naturally powerless to affect our health to any great degree. In fact, this couldn't be further from the truth. The belief that DNA dictates the entire destiny of our cells is not true.[6]

During the late 1980s, coinciding with the launch of the Human Genome Project, the findings of revolutionary research led scientists to begin to develop a new view of how our cells function. These findings are the foundation of the science of epigenetics, which is challenging the traditional views of biology and medicine.[7]

Genes contain instructions that tell individual cells how to specialize themselves, such as whether to become a heart cell or a brain cell, and what functions to perform. However, genes by themselves do not control the body. Research has determined that environmental signals—which include our thoughts, feelings, and emotions—are the primary regulators of our genes. Our cells read and respond to the conditions of their environment by activating different protein switches. The switches that are activated regulate the activity of the genes and control cell behavior. Remarkably, the same genetic blueprint has the capacity to create an excess of 30,000 variations of proteins, which are the body's molecular building blocks.[8]

The new understanding of our biology includes the fact that perception plays a role in genetic activity. You're already controlling your genes. Now and always, your mind and your lifestyle have been continuously influencing their expression.

YOUR FLEXIBLE GENES

At the end of every strand of DNA is a caplike structure called a *telomere* that prevents the aberration or loss of genetic information during cell division. Cell division is how your cells replicate and replace themselves throughout your life span. Your telomeres play a key role in maintaining the stability of your genetic codes. They are long when you are born, but each time your cells divide, the process causes your telomeres to shorten. Only a certain number of replications are possible before this happens, for every time a cell replicates itself, the gene becomes slightly less perfect; that is, your cells are being degraded as you grow older. Over the course of a lifetime, after the telomeres reach a critically short length, usually during the later years of life, your cells will develop the inability to divide again and begin to die without replacement. So they are now considered important markers of aging, chronic disease, and mortality.

A key question under investigation by researchers is whether there is any way to prevent or reverse the shortening of telomeres. Your telomeres are affected by many factors, including your cellular environment. It's been demonstrated that stress can accelerate telomere shortening and lead to early cellular aging. Telomere length reflects not only the presence of stress but also your body's response to it at a cellular level. Shortened telomere length is linked to aging, cancer, and heart disease.[9]

To reiterate: Our DNA is not the ultimate determinant of our health. For decades we were led to believe that our family genetic inheritance is the best indicator of our future state of health, but we now know better. Our lifestyle—in particular, our emotional lifestyle—plays a significant role in maintaining the health of our cells and organs.

Epigenetics has revealed that our internal environment of thoughts, feelings, attitudes, and emotions; our lifestyle, including what we eat; and our external environment all affect our genes. These factors have the ability to turn on and off the genetic codes that are responsible for either improving our health or making us more susceptible to disease.

Molecular biologist Elizabeth Blackburn won the 2009 Nobel Prize in Physiology as a result of her research determining that positive lifestyle changes (in particular, successful stress management) can reverse telomere shortening. Dr. Blackburn identified the enzyme telomerase, which maintains telomere length, while investigating the theory that psychological stress alters the rate of cellular aging. Her research on women determined that those with the highest levels of perceived stress had much shorter telomeres than those with lower levels of perceived stress.[10]

It is clear that epigenetic factors affect both our short-term and long-term responses and are key in determining how well our telomeres function. Recent studies have revealed that telomeres are powerful indicators of life's great insults. They are shortened by exposure to significant abuse in childhood, and they are shortened even more each year an individual spends depressed, caring for a sick loved one, going through a bankruptcy or a divorce, and so on. Most people are living with one or more ongoing life stressors resulting from their work, relationships, and world events.[11]

Your emotional response to stressful situations, especially to anything you perceive as a threat, can lead to a prolonged state of physiological arousal, a heightened fight-or-flight response that may affect cell longevity. A perception of threat—or even a cycle of negative thinking—triggers a cascade of negative emotional responses that intensify the significance of whatever seems threatening, making its presence seem even more stressful. Accelerated telomere shortening is linked to stressful life circumstances, psychological distress, aging, and disease. It is even associated with pessimism.[12]

Several studies involving men ages twenty-seven to sixty-five with mood disorders, increased stress, poor self-rated mental health, childhood trauma, and cognitive impairment and decline were found to have shorter telomere lengths compared to other men of the same ages.[13] Pessimism was the first personality trait to be linked to shorter telomere length.[14]

THE DEEP CONNECTION BETWEEN STRESS AND DISEASE

If you are to activate your internal superhealing power and deal adequately with your stress, it is critical for you to gain control of your thoughts and emotions. I cannot overstate how important it is to master your emotions. All of my clinical and personal experiences have persuaded me that no other factor is more beneficial to your health. Not diet, not exercise, and not even a good night's sleep will effectively reduce or eliminate your stress as much as altering your perception of stressful situations does. It is as significant as the discovery of the importance of hand washing in preventing bacterial and viral infections by surgeon Joseph Lister in the late 1800s, which completely changed the face of modern medicine and has saved millions of lives.

Stress is a state of mind that is a unique experience for each person. It reflects our responses not only to major life events but also to the conflicts and pressures of daily life that change our physiology. When stress is chronic, it is like a constantly ringing alarm system.

It burns through our critical energy reserves, overuses our key hormones, and leads to the depletion of our cellular resources. At least 85 percent of all illnesses, especially the most common ones (e.g., cancer, diabetes, high blood pressure, stroke, and asthma) are related to stress.[15]

The burden that stress puts on the body is related not only to life experiences but also to genetic differences and lifestyle. Epigenetic factors during childhood—including diet, physical activity, sleep, and emotional well-being—set lifelong patterns of reactivity and behavior through biological embedding. A 2011 study of long-term patterns of stress and their effect on longevity determined that individuals with moderate and high stress died at a younger age than those with low stress.[16]

The major challenge caused by stress is disruption of the body's internal balance. Chronic stress makes it virtually impossible to maintain homeostasis. Much akin to the burning of rubber on a spinning tire trapped in mud, the stress response is triggered by ongoing and unresolved anxiety, fear, tension, anger, and sadness. Besides causing noticeable changes in the body, such as increased heart rate, muscle tension, and hyperalertness, it shuts down the digestive and immune systems. Over long periods of stress, the body's ability to ward off infection is weakened. Stress chemicals also cause inflammation, which contributes to the development of numerous disorders.[17]

Any kind of emotional stress can impair your immune system, especially when the stress is severe or lasts for a significant amount of time. But even relatively short stressful periods, such as final exam week for a college student, can suppress immunity. The types of life stressors that could render you more vulnerable to disease include marital conflict and divorce, long-term unemployment, and work-related issues.[18]

After exposure to stress, certain hormones are released by the adrenal glands to help the brain return to its normal functioning.[19] But when the intensity or duration of stressors exceeds a certain threshold, which is unique for each person, the release of stress hormones can damage the brain and the rest of the body.[20] Chronic stress causes profound changes in human behavior, including anxiety, symptoms of depression, learning impairment, and memory loss.[21] At the same time, actual damage occurs to certain portions of the brain, and the ends of the nerve cells, which connect to other nerve cells, are impaired.[22] These changes primarily occur in the hippocampus, the part of the brain that plays an important role in memory, emotions, and cognition. A loss of volume in the hippocampus is associated with chronic diseases like Alzheimer's, heart disease, and diabetes.

According to Dr. Blackburn, "We tend to forget how powerful an organ the brain is in our biology." In an interview published in the *Atlantic*, she noted, "It's not that you can wish these diseases away, but it seems we can prevent and slow their onset with stress management."[23]

Positive and negative emotions are associated with a variety of immune system components. I'm focusing on what happens when we're distressed, because that's how most of us are, at least some of the time, and we probably don't know how to stop.

"What's making you sick?" is a question I ask patients during their initial visit to me. Although I originally thought that most people were unaware of their stress, I have since found that a surprising 95 percent of people will answer the question immediately by saying, "I'm living with a lot of stress." Rarely is there a disconnection in their minds between the stress that is occurring in their lives and their physical health.

I'd like to ask you a similar question now for your consideration before you go on reading. What's interfering with your experience of optimal health and well-being? Awareness is the first key ingredient to tapping into your mind's superhealing abilities. When you are able to answer this question truthfully, you will create a space in your mind that aligns you with your superhealing power.

This is indeed a marvelous time for those of us who decide to take charge of our health and well-being. The information available today is nothing short of remarkable. The research on how our minds and bodies interact inspires me. Years ago I set out on a path to improve my health and well-being, and I remain on that path to this very day. For a long time, I focused exclusively on my physical health. Then, during a hospitalization for a heart condition, I realized how deeply I was being affected by my emotions, and I began to pay more attention to the health of my mind. I learned to manage my thoughts, and I am now happy to report that I no longer experience the heart problem.

The body-mind-spirit whispers, speaks, and screams its messages to us about what it needs, and it slaps us down if we don't listen. When I ask the people I coach about their health the simple question "What's stressing you?" most answer without missing a beat. They are aware of what's causing their stress, but they usually feel helpless to address their responses to it, because they believe they have little or no control over their emotions. Fortunately, this can be changed. Our seemingly knee-jerk stress-induced emotional responses can be reined in and transformed.

YOUR UNFOLDING BRAIN: NEUROPLASTICITY

Colleen (not her real name) experienced a devastating stroke that paralyzed the left side of her body. I watched her valiantly struggle to relearn how to walk and incrementally recover. In the beginning, her physicians feared she wouldn't live, much less recover. Her family maintained a close watch over her as she improved. I wondered if she'd ever walk again, but her persistence and commitment allowed her to regain her ability to walk. At one time, it was believed that a stroke caused permanent damage, but now we know that the brain can reorganize itself. She did really well, valiantly and actively recovering from a stroke that paralyzed the left side of her body. In a few weeks, her brain reprogrammed itself, creating new pathways that bypassed the damaged area that had controlled her ability to move her left arm and leg.

Did you know that your brain has the ability to regenerate? For most of the twentieth century, the prevailing scientific opinion among neuroscientists was that brain structure is fixed and unchangeable after childhood. In medical school, my fellow students and I were taught that nerve cells were different from other cells because they lacked the ability to regenerate. Now we know that this simply isn't true. In recent decades, a vast array of research has revealed that the brain remains plastic—adaptive and moldable—even into adulthood.[24] Scientists have proved that the brain has a dramatic capacity to change in response to stimulation throughout every stage of life. In particular, the discovery that the adult brain can create new cells, a phenomenon known as *neurogenesis,* has caused a major shift in medical protocols and given us a new appreciation of our capabilities.[25] The concept of neuroplasticity has replaced the formerly held position that the brain is a physiologically static organ.[26]

Our brains change in response to our experiences in a multitude of measurable ways, from the growth of new connections between existing nerve cells to the birth of new cells. The brain is, in fact, so exquisitely responsive to shifts in our thinking, feeling, emotions, and behavior and to the external environment that we should take this as encouragement to purposefully continue to grow, learn, and develop new skills and talents for our entire life spans. The brain is far more dynamic than most people realize. It is never too late to change. This process is actively involved in how we change our response to distress.

Neuroplasticity occurs on a variety of levels, from cellular changes caused by learning to the large-scale changes of cortical remapping in response to injury. The role of neuroplasticity is widely recognized in healthy development, learning, memory, recovery from brain damage, and the successful management of stress.

Your brain's plasticity is important because that determines how efficiently your brain works. The more connections your brain makes, the easier it is for you to process information and make decisions. During your lifetime, your brain's capabilities will increase and decline depending on your lifestyle. Use them or lose them.

By seeking to determine the outer limits of the brain's capacity, scientists discovered that we can change the brain's structure by altering our thought processes—our beliefs. Do you realize how profound the implications of this are for your health and well-being?

We know now that the brain is a relay station of sorts. Our thoughts are not just words, impressions, and pictures floating through our heads, they are chemical and biological messengers that can and do affect the pathways they move through. The connection between our cognition and our physical condition is so profound that if we learn to manage our thoughts, feelings, and emotions, we can harness them to treat physical and mental disorders and deepen our sense of spiritual connection.

We can use the power of the mind to enhance our capacity to experience and express anything, including love, empathy, gratitude, and compassion.

THE POWER OF YOUR BELIEFS

Your beliefs have the power to change your physiology and improve your health. They also have the power to harm you. As demonstrated by the perceptual and emotional stimulation of your stress response, your beliefs can unleash very powerful forces inside your body.

My most intense personal experience with the extraordinary power of belief came when I was part of a team of doctors treating George (not his real name), who for several months had been experiencing unusual pain and other symptoms in his intestinal tract. A soft-spoken man in his late sixties, he had been referred to our hospital because his local doctors could not diagnosis the cause of his symptoms.

Throughout his diagnostic tests, George was quiet, cooperative, and extremely pleasant. After several days, an unfortunate diagnosis of terminal pancreatic cancer was made. I was in his room when his physician gave him the news, surrounded by our entire medical team. George looked as though a bomb had exploded in his mind. Stunned and unable to respond, he sat before us in a stupor. He didn't ask any questions. His wife, who was at his side, seemed more engaged. An hour or so later, she stopped me in the hallway just outside her husband's room. She grabbed my hand, looked directly into my eyes, and asked, "Is my husband going to die?"

Since her husband's primary physician had already told them he would die, I knew in my heart that she was searching for a ray of hope that I couldn't provide. Her sincerity pierced my heart. I wasn't equipped to answer the question, so I stumbled through with a response that neither comforted nor soothed her. "We're all going to die one day. I don't think anyone knows exactly when that's going to happen." I didn't know what else to say. With that, I awkwardly escaped her grip and went about my business. Looking back on that scene, I now wonder if perhaps George's wife had felt something in her husband's response that caused her more concern than the doctor's words.

After lunch, I walked past George's room and noticed that a nurse was changing his sheets. The room was empty. I wondered where he and his wife were. I didn't think any additional diagnostic tests were scheduled, so I asked the nurse. She replied, "George just died."

I was stunned. I raced to the nurses' station and asked my intern if he knew what had happened. "Seems like he had a heart attack," he answered. "I'm not sure we'll ever know. Considering he was terminal, an autopsy really isn't in order."

I believe the news of George's diagnosis frightened him to death. I really do. There have been numerous reports of people receiving frightening news and dropping dead on the spot. The damaging changes to the brain that occur in the face of significant stress can be attributed to its adaptability to the environment. Our beliefs direct and shape our whole physiology in remarkable ways.

Perhaps the most significant example of the power of belief is the placebo effect. A placebo is an inert substance without any medicinal value, such as a sugar pill, that is given to a person who is under the false impression that it is an effective treatment. An individual's belief alone can sometimes prompt an improvement. *Placebo* is Latin for "I shall please." Thus, the *placebo effect* is the medical term used to describe the healing power of the mind.

Traditionally, even though the placebo effect can be measured, it is explained in a way that minimizes its true power. Among researchers, the placebo effect is presented as a nuisance, an interfering human artifact that compromises the pure approach of scientific research on active substances, such a medications and surgery. As a young doctor, I learned that the placebo effect was something we "just had to live with." It was to be tolerated, not accepted as a possibility in planning a course of treatment. However, I was absolutely fascinated by the notion that the mind was so powerful. Although most people have heard of the placebo effect, I do not think many of us appreciate the opportunity it represents.

Your beliefs are quite powerful and have a direct effect on your body's responses. In fact, under the right conditions, your mind can heal your body in the absence of drugs or surgery. This is one of the most fascinating aspects of your superhealing ability.

The placebo effect is recognized as being so potent that for any new drug to be considered a valid healing agent, it must be measured against a placebo to prove its effectiveness compared to the effectiveness of beliefs. To be approved by the Food and Drug Administration, every new drug study includes a placebo, and most approved drugs actually do only a little better than placebos. But doctors and drug companies don't generally advertise this fact. As Ted Kaptchuk, a Harvard University professor and researcher who has spent his career studying the effect of placebos, has said, "Mainstream medicine uses the placebo effect all the time. Doctors don't tell you the drug they're giving you is barely better than a placebo. They all spin."[27]

In drug studies that take into consideration the power of the mind, the statistical difference between the "real thing" and the placebo is rarely more than 15 percent. Several studies have proved that placebo-induced sham treatments produce outcomes equal to those attributed to drugs and surgery in terms of providing relief from several common conditions. For instance, at Baylor College of Medicine, a group of orthopedic surgeons led by J. Bruce Moseley were prompted to explore the true benefits of a type of arthroscopic knee surgery that is recommended to patients with osteoarthritis when medication fails to relieve their pain. Although the surgery brings results, it is unclear to surgeons what the true physiological source of pain relief is. There is no proof that arthroscopy actually cures or halts the process of osteoarthritis. So this team of surgeons designed a study to assess the true effectiveness of arthroscopic surgery.

The Baylor College study was a double-blind design, which means that neither the subjects nor the researchers themselves knew which patients received arthroscopic surgery and which did not. There were 180 patients with degenerative knee arthritis in the study; the experimental group was given one of two kinds of authentic orthopedic surgery—one using a laprascope, the other using lavage (washing out) or debridement (removal of tissue)—and the control group was given a fake surgery. In the control group, three scalpel incisions were made around the knee like those used in actual surgery so as to keep the patients and the medical evaluators from discovering that they hadn't been operated on. The results of all the surgeries—both of the real ones and the fake one—were the same. The findings determined that surgery mostly relieves pain because the patients believe it does.[28]

Knee surgery for arthritis is not the only operation to be undermined when compared with sham surgery. Another study found something similar with patients undergoing a common procedure called vertebroplasty, which involves an injection into the lumbar spine. The procedure alleviated pain to the same degree as a placebo "surgery" in which the physicians tapped on the spine and piped in the smell of cement to the treatment room to make groggy volunteer subjects believe they were receiving the real treatment. Researchers found that the thirty-six volunteers who received the sham surgery did just as well as the thirty-five who got the real operation.[29]

One of the most fascinating double-blind studies I've seen compared the placebo effect to neurosurgery for Parkinson's disease, a serious disorder marked by the brain's diminished ability to produce dopamine, the chemical that is released when we feel pleasure. The study found that those who received a real transplant of dopamine neurons experienced improvement in their movement, whereas those who had sham surgery did not. Even so—and this is the part that intrigues me—the participants' perception of having had surgery did influence their responses. In their report, the researchers stated, "Those who thought they received the transplant at twelve months reported better quality of life than those who thought they received the sham surgery, regardless of which surgery they actually received."[30] In other words, their beliefs improved their lives.

Researchers at the University of California at Los Angeles have also investigated whether brain activity is altered by placebos. Their study involved giving patients with major depression a placebo instead of an antidepressant drug while leading them to believe they were receiving the actual drug. Using an imaging technique known as quantitative electroencephalography, the researchers discovered that the brain function of those who received the placebo was quite similar to the brain function caused by the antidepressant drugs. After nine weeks, the patients were classified as being medication responders, placebo responders, or, in some cases, nonresponders to either medication or placebos. Among the participants who were responders, it was found that the same brain region was changed whether they were medication responders or placebo responders.[31]

The researchers didn't anticipate that the participants receiving the placebos would actually have detectable changes in the speed and processing of their brain functions, but they did.

The mind is so powerful that it has also been observed to exert a negative influence on patients who have been told that an inert substance might be harmful. This phenomenon is called the *nocebo effect*. I believe that physicians accidentally induce a nocebo effect by handing out pessimistic predictions to their sick patients like judges handing down death sentences in court. Patients can so easily internalize the hopelessness their doctors feel and turn it into a self-fulfilling prophecy. Fortunately, doctors are increasingly being trained in the role the mind plays in health and disease, so they know to avoid triggering negative perceptions in their patients.

The German Medical Association, it is interesting to note, actively encourages physicians to prescribe placebos. In 2010, it found that 59 percent of patients with stomach discomfort were helped by sham treatments.[32]

POSITIVE PSYCHOLOGY

I love psychology. I minored in it in college and for a while seriously considered becoming a psychiatrist because of my desire to learn about the mind. When I first heard about the pioneering work of psychologist Martin Seligman, a professor at the University of Pennsylvania, I wanted to get on a plane, find him, and embrace him. He has devoted his career to studying uplifting traits such as optimism, peace of mind, and happiness, which help us navigate life without mental and emotional impairment.

Establishing a positive emotional state is one of the foundations of superhealing, for it aligns the mind with the true nature of the spirit. "Cheerfulness is the best promoter of health," said writer Joseph Addison, "and is as friendly to the mind as to the body." The field of positive psychology studies how to create conditions for peak performance and emotional resilience. From time immemorial we've known that positive emotions are antidotes to problems associated with negative emotions. The approach of positive psychology is to understand the underlying mechanisms of coping and uplifting.[33]

Whenever we talk about positive and negative feelings, there are bound to be a lot of misconceptions. So I want to emphasize that it is important to be authentic about your feelings: Don't suppress or deny negative emotions, but don't dwell on them or get stuck in feeling bad. If you're feeling down, acknowledge it and work on generating a better feeling. Focus on the good. Just this one step can improve your quality of life and health. It is important to move in the direction of positive thinking because of the clear-cut physiological and psychological advantages, especially in the long run.

I've often heard the argument that optimistic people are acting like Pollyanna, a rather saccharine young orphan in a novel of the same name who had learned from her father, since deceased, to find something to appreciate in every situation. Some people view optimism as unrealistic and even delusional. Isn't it interesting that realism is perceived as synonymous with negativity or unhappiness, whereas a positive outlook is believed to be unreal?

Whether positive thinking is good for you largely has to do with the intentions you are expressing. If you are in denial or suppressing your feelings, you are not being honest with yourself. Until you resolve the issues that your negative emotions are signaling require your attention, being superficially positive will not serve you.

Your highly adaptive brain cells have the ability to develop new neural networks. Even if you are a pessimist or locked in the throes of chronic stress, by working every day to change the tone of your thoughts and emotions, you can improve your health and well-being. You can train your mind to be optimistic and also to identify the patterns of thought that lead you to feel stress so you can interrupt them.

One of the most powerful beliefs you can develop is an underlying conviction of your ability to successfully manage situations that you perceive as stressful or threatening. Positive beliefs like this will enable you to transcend negative experiences.

Positive emotions enhance our well-being. The emerging research indicates that finding ways to cultivate positive emotions is crucial to creating optimal physical and psychological well-being.[34] By their very nature, positive emotions are expansive, and I believe they are so because they are not only in harmony with but also reflective of our true spiritual nature. I believe that stress comes from our failure to perceive ourselves as we truly are: remarkable, extraordinary, intelligent beings with the internal resources to overcome even the most difficult circumstances and experiences.

We now know that very positive emotions interrupt the stress response. When we perceive ourselves as being in control of our situation, this helps the brain to determine whether a situation should be viewed as a threat or a challenge. Such determinations are the primary drivers of our response to stress. Feeling a lack of control, uncertainty, and unpredictability stimulates the release of cortisol, a stress hormone.[35]

Positive emotions broaden our thinking and enhance our mental flexibility and coping skills. Even temporary experiences of positive emotions can have lasting consequences. They give us a solid foundation upon which to allow the birth of new internal resources that will support our well-being on an ongoing basis. They also counteract the brain's innate tendency to engage in negativity, thus promoting internal balance, lowering the body's stress response, helping us recover from stress more rapidly, and granting greater functioning after stress.[36]

Positive emotions are also associated with greater longevity among people with heart disease and kidney disease.[37] Also, in the face of HIV/AIDS, a positive outlook can lead to measurable improvement of the condition.[38]

Having a grim or pessimistic view of the future, which means having an expectation of negative results or fewer positive results, has been shown to lead to earlier death and a more rapid progression of the diseases of aging, probably in part because of faster telomere shortening.[39] Being optimistic and expecting good things to happen relates to better health. Positive emotions help us to develop hardiness and resilience (the ability to transcend our challenges) when they are firmly grounded by self-awareness and acceptance. They allow us to not only survive but thrive.

LIVING WITH AWARENESS

Every day your genetic activity changes as a result of the way you are feeling. Your mind's perception is directly reflected in your biochemistry: Neuropeptides released by your nervous system respond to your interpretation of the environment. This regulates your cellular environment, which means you can actually change your physiology and alter your genes through the way you think and feel. Positive emotions activate our genes in ways that protect and improve our health, whereas negative emotions turn on genes that ultimately contribute to disease production.

Given this reality, what are the best thoughts to think and the best feelings to feel? The short answer is anything uplifting. You will best be able to sustain your health if you are self-aware (so you know when something is off and requires attention or intervention) and if you know how to focus inwardly to induce the relaxation response. Just as the processes of respiration, digestion, and reproduction work best when you are relaxed, your healing capacity functions best when you are relaxed.

Optimal health is a state of harmony and balance. Thus, all living things, including humans, are innately equipped to be self-sufficiently healthy. We differ from other living creatures in one important respect: Our ability to experience optimal well-being depends in part on our willingness to learn to use our emotional capacities positively.

Paying attention to your feelings and emotions, and taking the time to honestly experience them as soon as they come up, is at the heart of superhealing. Sometimes you're frightened, anxious, or distressed. You could also feel lonely, hurt, and tired. Remember that these emotions are normal. Suppressing or ignoring them is unnecessary and undesirable. It's healthiest to acknowledge your feelings and see what needs and desires they are informing you of and then, to the best of your ability, redirect your thinking to an emotion that feels better. To improve your health and well-being and create a strong immune system, you must accept and honestly express your feelings. Maintaining a positive emotional state prevents wear and tear on the body and helps you avoid serious, chronic imbalances that set the stage for illness.

Living authentically and with awareness is a principal component of superhealing. So although it may take time and patience to increase your self-awareness and learn to regulate your thoughts and emotions, it is possible—and well worth doing.

Thanks to numerous important research studies, we now know that stress is not the issue; your response to it is. If you change your perception of what a stressful situation means to you, your physiology changes, and the damaging effects no longer persist.

There are many indications that thoughts and emotions are the keys to health. The scientific evidence clearly shows that the choices we make in terms of our perceptions, attitudes, beliefs, and emotions affect the body's response. Our thoughts and emotions stimulate the release of hormones and neuropeptides, the body's chemical messengers, which enable the body to respond in a positive adaptive way to stress.

A belief is any repeated thought that has been accepted by your unconscious mind as true. Because beliefs trigger the release of the chemicals that affect the entire body, if you believe something, it becomes true for you. A positive outlook is therefore a very powerful tool in dissipating disease. If you face stress with the right attitude and avoid internalizing destructive emotions, you will improve your physiology.

Your mind and your body are integrated, forming a mind-body unit. Each of the 50 trillion cells composing your body is an intelligent reflection of your thoughts and emotions. You therefore have the capacity to express the biology of hope, the physiology of love, and the neurochemistry of joy. Just think about the last time you were happy. Wasn't it a wonderful experience to feel that happiness permeating your entire body? When you're feeling down, your cellular function is down. But when you're happy, you are actually creating chemicals that sustain your happiness on a cellular level. That's the superhealing mind at work.

In the next chapter, we'll take a look at remarkable mind-body tools you can use to engage your superhealing mind.

CHAPTER 3

ENGAGING YOUR SUPERHEALING MIND

We are what we think.

All that we are arises with our thoughts.

With our thoughts we make the world. . . .

Your worst enemy cannot harm you

As much as your own thoughts, unguarded.

—*The Dhammapada*

YOUR MIND IS THE DOORWAY TO YOUR NATURAL SUPERHEALING ability. Since your thoughts and emotions are reflected in your physiology on a moment-to-moment basis, it is critical to uplift yourself mentally and emotionally. Fortunately, there are many ways to do this.

You do not have to passively experience your thoughts and feelings even though it may seem that you're at the whim of your moods and particularly the "voice" in your head. The same applies if your inner state veers toward the negative when you're under pressure or confronting difficult circumstances such as a disaster or an illness. Emotions follow thoughts, and there is much you can do to transform your thoughts to be more positive. The best place to begin is by making the conscious decision to do whatever is necessary to feel better than you do.

Do you remember the last time you felt anxious or angry? Did this feeling come on suddenly or grow in intensity? Was there a moment just beforehand in which something happened or was said that triggered you to have this experience? We can often sense ourselves

73

beginning to shift moods, and such moments are opportunities to pause and intervene. Make a decision that you will deliberately respond to the stresses and emotional triggers in your life in as self-nurturing a manner as possible and as soon as you can, and you'll be more resilient. As the evidence presented to you in the last two chapters indicates, this is a key to health.

We're healthier when we regularly engage in relaxation and laughter, condition our minds to seek and focus on positive outcomes, and find less harmful ways to express our challenging emotions. None of the techniques shared in this chapter are hard to do. If anything, the hardest part of engaging your superhealing mind, at least initially, is making it a habit to do so. Feeling better than you do right now is not an all-or-nothing proposition. It's a process for responding to life that moves you incrementally toward optimal wellness.

The more you practice engaging your superhealing mind, the better you will feel. The better you feel, the more the habit will be reinforced.

MAKING THE DECISION TO SUPERHEAL

Remarkable changes can occur, physiologically and psychologically, when you make a decision to engage your superhealing mind. These changes include everything from better sleep, fewer aches and pains, increased mental clarity, and improved memory to weight loss, lower blood pressure, more energy and stamina, and the reversal of chronic or life-threatening diseases. The mind regulates the brain and the nervous system, the endocrine system, the digestive system, the cardiovascular system, and every other system in the body. By engaging your mind in specific ways to reduce its perception of stress and the physiological affect it has on those systems, you can expand your capacity to heal and move toward optimal well-being.

In 1993, when I was teaching mind-body medicine to graduate

students in the Foundations of Holistic Health Program at DePaul University, southern Illinois was ravaged by floods that cut a wide swath across the state as the Mississippi River and other rivers overflowed. A state of emergency was declared. The assignment I gave my students was as follows: You are a volunteer on a mission to help the people affected by the floods—in particular, those who have lost their homes and livelihoods. You have no resources other than those you carry within your mind. Devise a program that will help them to effectively cope with this devastating experience. (Hint: Mind-body techniques are the key.) They created programs primarily composed of mind-body techniques that addressed the trauma of the experience and the emotional and spiritual needs of the affected people.

A decade later, I was pleased to discover that James Gordon the director of the Center for Mind-Body Medicine at the Georgetown University School of Medicine, was operating on the same wavelength. In 2007, after Hurricanes Katrina and Rita, he and other volunteers trained healthcare-professional survivors in several mind-body techniques to help them overcome the post-traumatic stress symptoms caused by these storms. The healthcare workers experienced compassion fatigue from helping others while they were coping with their own symptoms, which included insomnia, hyperalertness, and difficulty focusing. Ninety days later, the participants had improved: their symptoms were reduced, and their exhaustion, anxiety, anger, and depression had diminished. Dr. Gordon has also shared these techniques in conflict zones and other disaster areas around the globe.[1]

Mind-body techniques are growing in popularity and gaining a foothold in medical practice as the research conducted in the last forty years allows doctors to better understand their benefits. The techniques are powerful yet easy to do, inexpensive, and cost-effective, and they require little in the way of equipment. Furthermore, if you select several techniques and use them frequently, they will have a synergistic affect on your health. I myself now use mind-body techniques so often that they no longer even seem like special techniques to me; they are simply part of my daily routine.

THE POWER OF CONSCIOUS DECISION MAKING

There is a difference between responding to life by making choices, a mental process that requires us to expend energy, and making decisions, which saves energy. In a 2011 study of high-level cognitive processes, such as setting intentions and making decisions, the brains of the participants were scanned by magnetic resonance imaging (MRI) as they planned, previewed, and then executed one of three possible hand actions. In the planning phase, electromagnetic brain activity was significantly higher than it was after a decision was reached.[2] This indicates that the decision on how to pursue an intention brings a kind of ease in its wake. The internal resolution of making a conscious decision about our behavior sets us on course to pursue that intention without the need to expend time or energy revisiting or debating the issue.

Your first step in engaging your superhealing mind is to make a decision. The second step is to set an intention of how to do so. The techniques in this chapter can form the basis of your low-stress lifestyle once you decide to use them. At the end of the book, I will take you through the process—decide, intend, focus, and act—of creating your personalized superhealing action plan.

SUPERHEALING MIND ENGAGEMENT
TECHNIQUE #1: LAUGHTER

Are you surprised that I'm beginning with laughter? I am doing so because it is one of the easiest and yet most potent things you can do to enhance your well-being. "Always remember to laugh," Lord Byron once said. "It is the cheapest medicine." A hearty laugh, the kind that sends a stream of tears from your eyes, does more than warm the soul: it heals your body. Research has shown that laughter causes the lining of blood vessel walls, the endothelium, to relax, increasing blood flow for up to forty-five minutes after you laugh. Damage to the endothelium can lead to the narrowing of blood vessels and eventually the development of cardiovascular disease (atherosclerosis, the hardening of the arteries). That's no laughing matter—or maybe it is, since laughter prevents and even reverses this dangerous condition.[3]

When was the last time you had a really good, thigh-slapping belly laugh? Awhile back, I had too much to do. I was becoming more and more stressed, and I didn't have the time to take care of myself. When I did, I would go to sleep. One day, my stress got the better of me. While preoccupied with stressful thoughts, I failed to pay attention to where I was walking and inadvertently sprained my ankle. That evening, I laughed for a good solid hour, if not longer, while watching a funny movie at home with my husband, Victor. When the movie was over, my swollen and aching ankle didn't hurt anymore. I hadn't noticed it for the entire duration of the film. This experience was a powerful reminder of the role that laughter can play in superhealing. Since then, I've threatened to become a comedian for my next career! I've always enjoyed a good laugh.

A continually expanding body of medical research recognizes the benefits of laughter in preventing and reversing disease caused by the effect of stressful events on our lives. The medical world has studied humor and found that mirthful laughter, the type of laughter associated with humor, positively affects most of the body's major systems: circulatory, respiratory, muscular, nervous (including the brain), endocrine, and immune.[4]

The stimulation that laughter provides improves circulation because of its effects on the heart and the blood pressure. It helps the lungs to process oxygen more efficiently and improves the conditioning of the heart muscle. It also decreases the level of stress hormones circulating in the bloodstream and reduces muscle tension and pain. William Fry, now a professor emeritus at Stanford University, has conducted extensive research on the effects of laughter and concluded that several minutes of intense mirthful laughter is comparable to exercising for ten to fifteen minutes on a stationary bike or a rowing machine.[5]

Laughter is a happy, pleasant experience that alters our emotional response to stress. It temporarily shifts our attention, allowing us to experience the lighter side of life even in the face of adversity or illness. It enables us to release painful emotions like anger, fear, and boredom. Through laughter, we can leave behind crying and feeling like a victim, instead moving toward health and feeling like a survivor.

The ability to appreciate humor can reduce the mood disturbances that are the response to negative life events. Psychologically, it somehow gives us a greater sense of control over our lives. Although we cannot control the outside world and the things that happen in it, we do have the ability to control how we view these events and how we respond to them emotionally.

There is an interesting difference between the effects on our health of appropriate and inappropriate humor. The basic rule is that appropriate humor is inclusive: it brings people together. Any humor that is exclusive—that separates, offends, or lacks consideration of the feelings of others—is inappropriate. Therefore, it's no surprise to me that medical research has determined that appropriate humor is beneficial, whereas inappropriate humor is not.[6]

Superhealing Laughter Engagement Suggestions

The Association for Applied and Therapeutic Humor defines therapeutic humor as "any intervention that promotes health and wellness by stimulating a playful discovery, expression, or appreciation of the absurdity or incongruity of life's situations."[7]

Laughter is an effective self-care tool. It improves the body's function. Yet it is not merely a tool to be employed when you're stressed or unwell; it a gift of your humanity to be thoroughly enjoyed every day of your life. We're born laughing. Babies begin to laugh during the first few months of life. On average, children laugh about 150 times a day, whereas most adults laugh only 15 times a day. [8] Laughing will help you to stay young at heart.

Stronger social bonds are formed when laughter is shared.[9] Have you ever "caught" someone else's boisterous laughter? Surely you have! Nothing beats the feeling that comes from being "infected" like this. Laughter definitely helps us raise our happiness quotient.

To bring more smiles and laughter into your life, try one of these humor strategies:

1. Consciously intend to laugh.
2. Identify what types of things you find funny.
3. Cultivate a playful attitude.
4. Learn to tell jokes.
5. Create your own verbal humor.
6. Look for humor in your daily life.
7. Laugh at the silly things you do.
8. Purposefully find humor in the midst of stress.
9. Hang out with people who make you laugh.

Let's start laughing!

SUPERHEALING MIND ENGAGEMENT
TECHNIQUE #2: MEDITATION

Like laughing, many of the techniques I am sharing with you in this book come naturally to us as children. For instance, I used to meditate in my closet as a child—although I didn't call it that back then. My parents gave me and my sister, Denise, a cartoon slide projector when I was six or seven years old. We soon discovered that the darkest space in our house was the closet in our bedroom. One day, after we had completed our viewing, I remained behind. For some reason, the enveloping darkness caught my attention once I had turned off the projector. I loved it. I sat still in the velvety darkness and quiet, and it brought me peace. Hiding out in the closet became a routine after that. Whenever I emerged from my "escape pod," I felt refreshed.

The word *meditation* is derived from the Latin verb *meditari,* meaning "to think over, contemplate, reflect, consider, or ponder." The root of this Latin verb, *med,* which means "to measure," is also the root of the English word *medical.*[10] Until recently, the practice of meditation has been almost exclusively limited to the confines of the world's major religions. However, meditation doesn't necessarily have to be tied to any religious practice. It is currently one of the most popular mind-body techniques in the United States. In 2007, nearly 9.4 percent of adults, more than 20 million people, reported meditating within the past year.[11]

In general, meditation is any conscious mental process that induces the set of physiological changes known collectively as the *relaxation response.* During the 1970s, Harvard University researchers, led by noted cardiologist Herbert Benson, documented that meditation causes a state of profound rest by instigating a calming effect on the human body.[12] Meditation facilitates psychological coping and superhealing through relaxing the body and other physiological changes that are governed by the hypothalamus.

One of the most memorable studies Dr. Benson did became the subject of an ABC documentary in 1985.[13] He videotaped Tibetan monks in a monastery in the mountains of northern India drying cold wet sheets with their body heat. The loincloth-wearing monks sat quietly in a cold room where the temperature was only a few degrees above freezing. Using a meditation technique known as *g Tum-mo*, they entered a state of deep relaxation and meditation. Other monks soaked three-by-six-feet sheets in cold water (forty-nine degrees Fahrenheit) and wrapped them across the shoulders of the meditating monks.

Even when wearing clothes, most humans experience uncontrollable shivering at this temperature. It can quickly cause hypothermia, a condition in which the body's temperature is too low to support organ function, and it rapidly causes death. Because of their meditation training, however, the monks didn't shiver. I couldn't believe my eyes! A thick cloud of steam rose from the sheets that required the cameraman to repeatedly wipe off his camera's lens in order to continue filming.

The Dalai Lama permitted Benson and his team of researchers to measure the monks' physiology while in the deep states of meditation. They were astonished to find that these monks could lower their metabolism by 64 percent. Dr. Benson noted, "Buddhists feel the reality we live in is not the ultimate one. There's another reality we can tap into that's unaffected by our emotions, by our everyday world. Buddhists believe this state of mind can be achieved by doing good for others and by meditation. The heat they generate during the process is just a by-product of g Tum-mo meditation."[14]

In our society, meditation is commonly used to reduce stress, cope with illness, and enhance overall health and well-being. Various meditative practices have been linked with positive outcomes, including improved functioning in the areas of mood, compassion, self-control, self-esteem, academic achievement, concentration, and memory.[15] Research findings also indicate a positive correlation with reductions in stress, anxiety, depression, headaches, pain, blood pressure level, and more. Researchers at the University of Massachusetts and Massachusetts General Hospital, found that those who meditated approximately half an hour per day during an eight-week period reported at the conclusion of the study that they were better able to function with heightened awareness and non-judgmental observation, more empathy, introspection and the ability to consider the viewpoint of others.[16]

How Meditation Works

Today we know that the relaxation response can be stimulated by various techniques that cause relaxation: meditation, visualization, biofeedback, hypnosis, progressive relaxation, and controlled breathing. All of these trigger the relaxation response by interrupting our normal thought patterns to focus on something else—the breath, a word, a phrase, a prayer, an object—while easing our ongoing involvement with our stream of thought. The components of meditation are a self-induced state of physiological relaxation, a shift of awareness, self-observation, and concentration.[17] Meditation is effective because relaxation is a result of the sympathetic nervous system's reduced activity and the parasympathetic nervous system's increased activity.[18]

Molecular biologist Jon Kabat-Zinn the founder of the Mindfulness-Based Stress Reduction Program at the University of Massachusetts Medical Center, teaches an approach to meditation based on incorporating mindfulness, or moment-by-moment nonjudgmental awareness. Various techniques are used to help the participants become more aware of their bodies, thoughts, and emotions in the present moment. These include scanning the body, letting one's thoughts arise and pass, and being aware of the taste and texture of the food one is eating.[19]

Research indicates that in addition to reducing stress and its physical symptoms, mindfulness meditation leads to positive emotions and improves quality of life. Practicing this meditation affects your mind, brain, body, and behavior in ways that promote whole-person health. The benefits of a mindfulness practice include an increase in the body's ability to heal and a shift from a tendency to use the right prefrontal cortex to a tendency to use the left prefrontal cortex. This shift is associated with relieving depression and anxiety and enhancing relaxation and well-being.[20]

There is also a relationship between the amount of time we spend practicing meditation and the intensity of the positive effects it has on our mental and physical health.[21] In other words, the more you do it, the healthier you become. Many religions utilize meditative techniques such as contemplation, affirmation, and prayer. Research shows that when we combine such practices with faith-based beliefs, it intensifies their positive effect on our health and well-being.[22]

Some researchers have argued that certain meditative practices are more effective than others. The good news is that they are all effective. Although some do affect brain functioning differently and may offer particular cognitive benefits that kick in after years of practice, all provide similar health benefits.[23]

For the purpose of your own superhealing, feel free to choose whichever type of meditation you prefer—you can even use more than one technique, if you like.

Superhealing Meditation Engagement Suggestions

In my medical practice, I encourage my patients to take simple steps to meditate, and I teach several basic meditative practices. (Find a free healing meditation to begin with at my website, http://www. drelaine.com/healingmeditation). Some patients choose to focus on breathing, others select a word or an object to focus on, and still others simply let the mind rest. Whatever you choose, focus and awareness are the key elements.

According to the National Center for Complementary and Alternative Medicine, most types of meditation have four elements in common: a quiet space, focus, a comfortable posture, and open-mindedness.[24]

It is important to set aside a time to meditate and disconnect from the world. First thing in the morning is a good time because your mind has not completely returned to its normal waking state. Turn off your phone, television, radio, computer, and so forth and find a quiet place where you will not be interrupted. Some people create a meditation room or corner in their home. You can choose to meditate in silence or put on some gentle, meditative music. Just do what is comfortable for you.

SUPERHEALING MIND ENGAGEMENT TECHNIQUE #3: VISUALIZATION

"The soul . . . never thinks without a picture," Aristotle said. Visualization, the use of mental imagery to induce physiological changes, is another ancient technique that has reemerged in the contemporary world as a powerful healing tool.[25] This superhealing technique has gained acceptance among psychologists, teachers, athletes, and businesspeople and has filtered into mainstream modern medicine in the same way that meditation has. Often used in conjunction with prayer and meditation, visualization has been practiced in cultures around the world—in Africa, the Americas, China, Tibet, India, and Europe—since the time of the Egyptian pharaohs.[26]

Visualization is the act of imagining a reality through creating mental pictures. But it is not only visual; imagery includes every other sense as well: physical sensation, sound, smell, and taste. It's an internalized experience that encompasses emotions, words, sounds, and even subtle bodily sensations. It also includes imagery through storytelling and metaphor. Everyone visualizes, and constantly. Whenever we think about anything, whatever we're imagining involves imagery. In one-fourth to one-third of the population, however, the imagery is so fleeting that the person is not even aware it's occurring. Yet even though it can be outside our range of conscious perception, it is the natural way that our minds code, store, and express information.

Visualization has been used for more than a century in the field of psychotherapy. In the 1920s, daydreams began to be used in therapy.[27] Carl Jung referred to the technique of visualization as the directed waking dream, the active imagination, and guided affective imagery.[28] There are two ways to visualize: in a normal state of mind or in a meditative state. Visualizing while meditating is deemed more effective. Either way, visualization includes generating a stream of thoughts you can hear, see, feel, smell, and taste. These thoughts are an inner, and often symbolic, representation of your experience or your desires. Purposeful visualization can be a doorway to your inner self and a way of observing your own feelings, ideas, and emotions. But it is more than that: it is a means of achieving well-being, of transforming and releasing yourself from mental distortions that may unknowingly be guiding your behavior and affecting your health.[29]

Imagery is a natural language and a major part of the nervous system. Since the 1980s, many clinical studies have determined that visualization is an effective component in the treatment of a vast range of illnesses.[30] Visualization can assist you in developing positive emotions and expressing spiritual qualities, such as hope, courage, patience, perseverance, love, and others that can help you cope with, transcend, or recover from almost any illness.[31] Imagery can help whether you have a headache or a far more serious condition. While engaging imagery, you can invoke the relaxation response and use it to reduce, modify, or eliminate pain. Imagery will also assist you in changing lifestyle habits that may be contributing to poor health.

Fifty years ago, two doctors and a psychologist developed a program for cancer patients using imagery to promote healing. They proved that the immune system could be enhanced by visualizing stronger white blood cells attacking and consuming cancer cells. In their first study of 160 patients, 19 percent had their cancers entirely eliminated, 22 percent went into remission, and those who eventually died lived twice as long as their predicted survival times.[32]

Guided imagery has been used by athletes in training to enhance motor (muscle) functioning. Research has found that thinking about moving a part of the body specifically stimulates the nerves in the muscles of that area.[33] Harvard Medical School neuroscientist Alvaro Pascual-Leone conducted a recent study in which he instructed a group of people to practice a five-finger piano exercise as fluidly as they could while trying to keep to a metronome's sixty beats per minute. For five days, they practiced for two hours a day. At the end of each practice session, a transcranial magnetic stimulation (TMS) test was conducted: a coiled device was placed on the crown of the head to measure the activity of the nerves located beneath the coil in the motor cortex region of the brain.

The TMS mapped how much of the motor cortex controlled the finger movements for the piano exercise. The scientists found that after the five days of practice, the part of the motor cortex that was devoted to the finger movements took over the surrounding areas.[34] This finding was in line with a growing number of discoveries that the greater use of a particular muscle causes the brain to devote more area to it.

The experiment was then extended by having another group of volunteers merely think about practicing the piano exercise. They played the simple piece of music in their heads, holding their hands still while imagining how they would move their fingers. Then they too sat beneath the TMS coil.

When the scientists compared the TMS data on the two groups— those who actually played the piano and those who merely visualized playing—they discovered a revolutionary idea: the ability of a thought to alter the physical structure and function of the brain. The TMS confirmed that the region of brain that controls the piano-playing fingers also expanded in the brains of the volunteers who merely imagined playing the music—the same way it had for the players.[35]

Visualization causes the reorganization of the brain and can even change the brain's physical structure. This type of research is a meaningful continuation of the studies reported during the 1980s and 1990s that confirmed the capacity of the mind to control and direct a wide variety of physiological responses.[36]

Guided imagery can be used to affect the particular functions of the white blood cells that play a significant role in the immune system's response to invading organisms. In a 1983 study at Michigan State University, the student volunteers learned to control very specific functions of certain white blood cells using visualization. It caused an average of 60 percent more of the neutrophils (germ-destroying white blood cells) to leave the bloodstream and enter the surrounding tissue.[37] A Harvard study found that relaxation and imagery increased IGA, a very important immune system protein. The practices also enhanced the T cell, or lymphocyte, function, another important component of the immune system.[38]

Gerald N. Epstein, a professor of psychiatry at Mount Sinai Medical School in New York, has used imagery ever since he took a trip to Israel several decades ago and met a traditional healer who taught him a visualization technique. He now uses imagery daily in his medical practice. He teaches residents and attending physicians how to use it and has conducted grand-rounds lectures at his hospital on it. He has reported dramatic results, from spontaneous healing of cancer to significant reduction in the healing time of fractures to notable improvements in a variety of diseases.[39]

Imagery involving emotional topics can stimulate appropriate, even dramatic, bodily responses. Preliminary evidence suggest that visualization can tone and strengthen muscles similar to the way exercise does; it activates the same parts of the brain. During a study in the 1940s, subjects were instructed to imagine lifting different weights, and their muscle tension increased with the weight of the imagined lift. [40]

One study that taught patients to visualize before surgery found that it helped them to recover faster and use less pain medication, and it reduced the formation of postoperative hematomas, a condition in which blood collects beneath the skin and in the muscles. Other studies have shown that when patients with hypertension visualized their blood vessels dilating, their blood pressure became much lower than it did in patients who used only a relaxation technique [41]

A stress-management program composed of visualization, breathing exercises, and coping skills was found to help men with prostate cancer prepare for surgery. It decreased their presurgical anxiety and improved their immune system functioning after surgery.[42] And researchers at the University of California at San Francisco taught a group of asthmatics how to visualize, which improved their breathing compared to a control group of patients who weren't taught the technique.[43]

Visualization has also been found to stimulate specific cells in the immune system to impede tumor growth, and that process reversed when the practice was stopped.[44] Aggressive visualization isn't as effective for some cancer patients with unresolved feelings of anger, hate, grief, or loss. When disease is a manifestation of suppressed emotional energy turned back on itself, it reinforces such denial.

Superhealing Visualization Engagement Suggestions

You can use visualization as part of your meditative practice, during your free moments, and throughout the day while you're engaging in your normal activities. Keep in mind that visualizing is more potent when you involve *all* your senses to make the picture more realistic.

SUPERHEALING MIND ENGAGEMENT TECHNIQUE #4: EXPRESSIVE WRITING

Our thoughts, feelings, and moods have an effect not only on the development of certain diseases but also on the ultimate course those diseases take. Therefore, any coping mechanisms we can develop to manage our moods and meet our psychological needs are of great benefit to us. Expressing ourselves in writing with the specific aim of releasing painful or conflicted thoughts and feelings is one such solution.

When I was eleven or twelve, I started keeping a journal. There was something exciting and magical about describing my activities and my feelings about the events in my life on paper. It was appealing to give immortality to my most important and intimate thoughts (at least that's what I thought I was doing). Then I enjoyed reading, reviewing, and reconsidering my experiences. Keeping a journal has been a constant part of my life ever since.

Twenty years ago, I discovered the scientific basis for the power of writing about our lives to make us feel good. At a health conference, I heard social psychologist James W. Pennebaker, then the chairman of the psychology department at Southern Methodist University in Dallas, Texas, talk about the events that had led him to begin research in a new area: the psychology of expressive writing.

The subject of Dr. Pennebaker's lecture was an incident in which he met a man who had recently confessed to a murder that he'd kept secret for several months. In spite of the fact that this man was facing spending the rest of his life in prison, he expressed relief from making his admission. Hearing this, Pennebaker wondered whether the relief the man felt translated into physiological changes. He constructed a study to determine the extent to which it is healthy to express suppressed, stored, unprocessed, and unresolved emotions through a technique he called *cathartic writing*.

His research consisted of having participants write for fifteen to twenty minutes a day for four consecutive days about emotionally challenging topics and experiences. At the completion of the study, everyone showed signs of increased immune system functioning, and these positive changes continued for up to six weeks. Even months later, the participants reported making fewer doctor visits for stress-related illnesses.[45]

In his book *Opening Up*, Dr. Pennebaker explained that holding back our emotions is challenging and a difficult physiological state to maintain. "Active inhibition means that people must consciously restrain, hold back, or in some way exert effort to not think, feel, or behave."[46] Repressing and holding in emotions, most often done unconsciously, can become so stressful that it adversely affects us.

Writing specifically to release mental images of trauma and emotional pain or conflict engages the superhealing mind more than noncathartic writing does. In another study, Dr. Pennebaker compared one group of college students who wrote about trauma with another group who wrote about trivial things, such as descriptions of their dorm rooms. Before the study, all the students in the study had visited the campus health clinic at similar rates. Afterward, the trauma writers' visits were half those of the others.[47]

Pennebaker did a similar study among worksite wellness program participants and got similar results. He concluded, "The degree to which writing or talking about basic thoughts and feelings can produce profound physical or physiological changes is nothing short of amazing."[48]

Most interesting is that an analysis of people writing about trauma indicated that those whose health improved to the greatest degree tended to use more words about positive emotions.[49] The increasing sense of insight after several days of writing was also linked to health improvement. Creating a coherent story while honestly expressing negative emotions made the writing process a healing event. It prompted changes in the autonomic nervous system and, like other techniques, lowered stress hormone levels and promoted relaxation. Dr. Pennebaker and colleagues also found direct physiological evidence that writing increases the level of disease-fighting lymphocytes circulating in the blood and even causes blood pressure to decrease.[50]

Investigators are unsure of the precise physiological mechanism

that makes expressive writing effective medicine. Until 1999, research in this area focused mainly on healthy individuals. Then
psychologist Joshua M. Smyth and colleagues studied the effects of
keeping a journal in individuals with asthma and rheumatoid arthritis. The study, which involved sixty-one asthmatics and fifty-one
people with rheumatoid arthritis, is probably the very first to use
standard clinical outcome measurements to examine how writing
about stressful events affects specific illnesses. The asthmatics who
finished the study experienced 19 percent average improvement of
their lung functioning, and the patients with rheumatoid arthritis
had a 28 percent reduction of their symptoms of arthritis.[51]

Dr. Smyth and his colleagues asserted, "We can do a good job with
medication, but we can do a better job if we also pay attention to people's psychological needs . . . very minimal psychological social interaction can have very substantial medical effects."[52]

Writing about this study, Dr. David Sobel made the point that if
the authors of the study had provided similar evidence about a new
drug, it probably would have been in widespread use within a short
time:

> *We would think we understood the "mechanism" (whether
> we did or not), and there would be a mediating industry to
> promote its use. Manufacturers of paper and pencils are not
> likely to push journaling as a treatment addition for the man-
> agement of asthma and rheumatoid arthritis. But the authors
> have provided evidence that medical treatment is more effec-
> tive when standard pharmacological intervention is combined
> with the management of emotional distress. Expressing nega-
> tive emotions, even just to an unknown reader, seems to have
> helped these patients acknowledge, bear, and put into perspec-
> tive their distress.* [53]

Expressive writing has many benefits. The following list is adapted from Pennebaker and from Kathleen Adams.[54] Expressive writing does the following:

- Helps us integrate and organize our complicated lives in a variety of ways
- Clears the mind
- Helps resolve traumas that stand in the way of important tasks
- Helps in acquiring and remembering new information
- Fosters problem solving and forces people to sustain their attention on a given topic for a longer amount of time
- Lowers the blood pressure and heart rate and benefits the immune system
- Improves lung function in asthmatics
- Improves joint mobility in rheumatoid arthritis

The research confirms William Shakespeare's advice in *Hamlet* (Act 1, Scene 3): "To thine own self be true." Being honest with ourselves on paper allows for the realization that we have the capacity to define every experience, regardless of the depths of emotional pain it may have caused us. Not only do we possess the psychological and spiritual wherewithal to survive all our experiences, we also possess the ability to heal and to thrive.

Superhealing Expressive Writing Engagement Suggestion

If you are ready to take on expressive writing, I'd recommend committing to writing about anything that is troubling you and your feelings about it for at least fifteen minutes a day for the next month.

SUPERHEALING MIND ENGAGEMENT TECHNIQUE #5: POSITIVE THINKING, OR AFFIRMATIONS

Until the end of the twentieth century, scientists believed the brain was different from the rest of the body and could not change or regenerate itself. Fortunately, today we know that the brain has a remarkable capacity to adapt. Our brains respond to cues from our environment—including our thoughts, feelings, and emotions—by altering their own structures and functions.

Just as we practice playing the piano to get better at it, if we repeatedly practice certain ways of thinking, we become better at those, too. Positive thoughts repeated over time can powerfully alter the brain. If you decide to change your thinking by regularly replacing your undesirable thoughts with more positive ones, the neural pathways in your brain that once processed your old way of thinking begin to atrophy, just as a muscle does when you stop using it.

The idea that the brain is adaptable was first introduced by psychologist William James in 1890, and it was soundly rejected by scientists who believed that the brain is rigidly mapped out, with certain parts controlling certain functions. They believed that if a part of the brain was damaged, its function was altered or lost. Of course, we now know they were wrong. The discovery of neuroplasticity, that our thoughts can change the structure and functioning of our brains throughout our life spans, was one of the most significant breakthroughs in the understanding of the brain that has ever occurred. Science has proven that the brain is endlessly adaptable and dynamic.

Neuroplasticity means that if you make the effort, your thinking can change, even when your thoughts are habitual and seemingly out of your conscious control. As you make a conscious effort to adopt a different attitude, the brain circuits that processed your old way of thinking begin to fade. This process provides the brain with the ability to alter and enhance its structure and processing, even for those with the severe neurological afflictions. People with significant medical conditions like cerebral palsy, paralysis, stroke, and mental illness have successfully trained other areas of their brains to compensate through repetitive mental and physical activities. When you engage in ongoing, frequent positive thought and positive activity, it can rewire your brain and strengthen brain areas that stimulate positive feelings.

If you don't believe in the power of positive thinking, you are not alone. Neither did I when I first heard about it. I was skeptical when I was introduced to the practice of repeating affirmations, such as "I am healthy, happy, and whole," to uplift my thinking. And guess what: They didn't work for me. It turns out that belief and emotional commitment to the affirmation you are repeating is an essential aspect of the technique. Gradually, over the years, I began to consider the effect of my negative thinking on my health. Massive, sometimes uncontrollable, fears had taken hold of me, and I recognized that my anxiety was affecting my health, at least indirectly. I tried affirmations again and saw a dramatic, positive improvement in my state of being.

Since I've begun to monitor my negative thoughts, I've become much more aware of their power to influence my moods and health. I am certainly not on "thought patrol," and I don't recommend paying attention to each and every thought you have, because that would be far too time-consuming. But I do think it is important for you to take stock of trends in your thinking. It's like the difference between watching a wave and and watching the tide. An individual wave can knock you down from time to time, but it's more important to know when the tide has shifted direction.

Now that we understand that our thoughts shape the brain's wiring and establish patterns, we can practice repeating beneficial thoughts until they become imprinted on our brains and in our unconscious minds. These repeated thoughts are affirmations.

Affirmations so powerful because over time, whatever we think about repeatedly sets up chemical, biological, and electromagnetic patterns in our minds and our bodies. Since these become habitual, our thoughts are critical to our health and well-being. Affirmations can be a very important tool in the transformation of your thinking.

Superhealing Affirmation Engagement Suggestions

Get a fresh notebook and spend a few minutes a day for the next forty days writing down your affirmations and feeling them. You can make the affirmations any time of day that you like.

Focusing on your health, on getting well, as often as possible is important, because your thoughts and emotions engage your super-healing mind and catalyze your body's ability to heal and regenerate. Here are some affirmations I want to share with you; use these or go ahead and design your own:

- I am healthy.
- I am superhealing.
- I am a superhealer.
- I am strengthening my mind, fortifying my body, and expanding my spirit.
- My mind has superhealing powers.
- I am tapping into my superhealing powers, and my body, mind, and spirit are improving each and every day.
- I am focusing on my body's amazing, superhealing powers.
- I intend to improve my health.
- I am superhealing now.

- I am superhealing my life now.
- I have the ability to superheal.
- My body was created to superheal and has optimal health and well-being.
- I can superheal my life.
- I am getting well faster now.
- I am healthy, happy, and whole.
- My health is improving more and more, and I am superhealing faster than I can imagine.
- My body is strong and remarkable.
- I am feeling better and better.
- I am getting stronger and stronger.
- I am so happy and grateful for all that is functioning in my body.
- I am grateful for my body.
- I love my body.
- All is well in my body.
- All is well in my mind.
- All is well in my spirit.

These affirmations may sound silly, but let me assure you, if you focus on them or similar ones for at least fifteen to thirty minutes a day you will see a profound shift.

Psychologists call the affirmation technique *cognitive behavioral programming*. You can call it whatever pleases you. Just know that if you use affirmations appropriately on a daily basis, saying and feeling them as though they are literally true, it will change the cells and organs in your body. Affirmations can help you get well faster if you're sick. If you're well, they can help you establish and sustain optimal health and well-being.

SUPERHEALING WORK SHEET:
ENGAGING YOUR SUPERHEALING MIND

Choose one superhealing mind technique to play with for the next week. You don't have to wait until you've read the entire book to begin to experience these benefits. Commit to just ten to fifteen minutes a day; that is sufficient to begin. Answer the following questions:

1. Are you actively using any of these superhealing mind-body techniques?
2. Do you want to add more?
3. Which ones do you find most appealing?
4. How much time do you want to commit?
5. Do you have any reservations?
6. How do you think you can shift your perspective?
7. How many techniques are you willing to try?

Part Two

YOUR
SUPER HEALING
BODY

CHAPTER 4

ESTABLISHING A SUPERHEALING ENVIRONMENT

Study nature, love nature, stay close
to nature. It will never fail you.

—Frank Lloyd Wright

FOR MOST OF MY LIFE, I WAS A CITY DWELLER. I GREW UP IN DETROIT, went to college in Providence, Rhode Island, and for many years lived near my workplace in Chicago with my husband, Victor. Ultimately, however, city dwelling began to take a toll on me. I became increasingly sensitive to the loud noises, congestion, and fast-paced energy of my urban surroundings. I often felt on edge and had difficulty sleeping. My health already suffered for a variety of reasons related to stress, and the urban environment offered me little relief. Although I felt torn about relinquishing the city lifestyle, with its easy access to stores, restaurants, entertainment, and Lake Michigan (which was a five-minute walk from our home), I reluctantly did. A few years ago, we moved to a rural town an hour's drive away from the heart of the city, and this move restored me mentally, physically, and emotionally. My husband and I now live in the midst of one of Mother Nature's forests, a setting filled with the most beautiful sights and sounds I could ever imagine. The only noises I regularly hear these days are the calls of geese, sparrows, robins, woodpeckers, bluejays, and cardinals. On our property, I am able to watch and participate in the subtle changes of the seasons that I missed in the city. And even though I still work in an office in the city, every evening I am eager to return home to this peace and restoration. In my heart I know that living surrounded by nature has added years to my life by improving my health and well-being. Nature is one of the keys to superhealing.

THE STRESS OF URBAN AND MAN-MADE ENVIRONMENTS

More than half of the world's population now lives in urban environments, and by 2050, at least 66 percent of the global population will be city residents, according to sociologists' predictions. Although there are advantages to city life, the sensory input we constantly receive in cities makes them stressful places to live. A German study found that the amygdala, an area of the brain involved in the stress response, was much more active among urban residents and that another area of the brain involved in regulating the stress response, the cingulated cortex, was more active in people born in cities. In other words, living in the city causes an overstimulation of the brain, making urban dwellers much more susceptible to stress-related physical and mental illnesses.[1]

Cities are stressful because they are man-made settings: They are crowded, noisy, and visually distracting and have lots of social activity. Although rural and suburban dwellers also live in man-made environments, they tend to be spread out more; cities, in contrast, tend to be constricted places, with buildings standing tall and tight together. Most have a shortage of open spaces and sunlight and lack meaningful signs of nature or the opportunity to interact with it. Just being in an urban setting like this interferes with our most basic mental processes. After a few minutes of exposure to a crowded street setting, the brain loses a portion of its capacity to remember, and people experience diminished self-control.[2] For these reasons, city residents are generally more stressed than those living in the suburbs or in the country.

There is, of course, no place on the planet anymore that has not been affected by the presence of people, but in cities, besides being more crowded together, we are typically exposed to higher levels of toxic chemicals and pollution. Most cities have a visible layer of smog in the air above them, which comes from the fumes of cars and trucks, factories, dry cleaners, construction work, and trash incinerators. Cities are filled with the waste products of homes and businesses. Wherever we live today, we are exposed to thousands of chemicals on a daily basis—and ironically, a great number of these come from the cleaning products we use.

There are two kinds of toxicity to be aware of. The first is acute toxicity, which is caused by a large single dose of a poisonous substance. The second is chronic toxicity, a low-level exposure that leads to a gradual buildup in the body. It is remarkable how well our bodies can process and eliminate chemicals. But sometimes the body simply cannot keep up with the environmental demands placed upon it.

The liver, kidneys, intestines, and skin are the four principal organs of detoxification. It is best to minimize our toxic exposure as much as possible to ensure that these organs can do their jobs effectively so there is less buildup of toxins over time and we remain healthy. I recommend that you pay attention to the following toxins:

- **Lead.** Although regulations have changed, lead used to be in gasoline and paint. Exposure comes from the bottom of our shoes, which pick up lead particles that are then tracked into our homes. Take your shoes off when entering your home to reduce this kind of contaminant exposure. Lead can also get into our drinking water when plumbing equipment and old fixtures begin to corrode.[3] Use a water filter to purify your tap water.

- **Fluoride.** Long added to toothpaste and water-supply systems to prevent cavities, on the recommendation of the American Dental Association, fluoride is, in fact, harmful. It reduces children's intelligence; penetrates the bones, where it causes hip fractures and osteoporosis; and has also been linked to cancer in young males.[4] To protect yourself, choose a toothpaste that does not contain fluoride, and again, use a water filter to purify your tap water.
- **Mercury.** A liquid element, mercury is commonly found in products like lightbulbs and thermometers. It is also released into the environment when coal is burned, which many American factories do. The trouble is that when mercury particles from the air settle into water, the mercury is transformed into a highly toxic pollutant, methyl mercury, which builds up in the fish and shellfish and gets into our food supply.[5] The Environmental Protection Agency issues annual advisories of which kinds of fish are safest to eat. You can find its most up-to-date recommendations online at http://www .foodsafety.gov.
- **Bisphenol A (BPA).** Found in polycarbonate plastic and epoxy resins, BPA is present mainly in food and beverage containers but also in plastic shopping bags, the air, dust, water, and dental amalgams used for fillings.[6] A surprising source is the thermal paper used to print store receipts. You can protect yourself from BPA primarily by not drinking beverages stored in plastic bottles and by washing your hands after you shop.[7]
- **Aluminum.** Exposure to aluminum can come through the foods we eat and the air we breathe. It is especially hazardous to older people and those with diminished kidney function.

Symptoms of aluminum toxicity include osteoporosis, dementia, and anemia, since aluminum interferes with the body's ability to absorb iron. Some antacids, antiperspirants, and immunizations contain aluminum and so should be avoided whenever possible. Read product labels carefully.[8]

- **Pesticides.** Although farmers want to ensure that their crops are not damaged by insects, and no one wants to be bitten by mosquitoes, many of the chemicals that are used to retard bugs that eat crops and bite people are known to cause cancer if they reach certain levels in our bodies. You can limit your exposure to pesticides by eating organic produce and refraining from the use of bug spray.

- **Cleaning supplies.** Some of the most harmful chemicals we are exposed to regularly are the ones we keep under the kitchen sink or in the hall closet. You can be certain a product is toxic if it says so on the warning label, but many dangerous cleaning supplies are not explicitly labeled. Products to be wary of include toilet bowl cleaners, window-cleaning solutions, disinfectants, floor cleaners, spot removers, and laundry detergents. Be suspicious of anything that dissolves dirt. Also be cautious about coming into contact with or breathing the fumes of ammonia, formaldehyde, and chlorine.[9] To protect yourself, make your own substitutes. Many effective homemade cleaning supplies use natural ingredients, and recipes for these can be found online. Search for phrases like *nontoxic cleaning supplies* and *green cleaning products.*

In addition to regular exposure to man-made chemicals and pollution, the contemporary lifestyle, which takes place indoors, is detrimental to our well-being. Most of us don't get enough exposure to natural light and its health-giving benefits. Remember how good you felt on the last bright sunny day? Sunshine affects my mood in a positive way. I can actually feel the light entering through my eyes and revitalizing my brain. It's hard for me to be anything other than happy and mentally alert on sunny days.

Although excessive exposure to sunshine has been linked to the development of certain skin cancers, the benefits of direct sunlight in appropriate doses of up to thirty minutes a day should override that concern. One of the most important benefits of sunlight is its stimulation of the skin to produce vitamin D. Research indicates that more than 1,000 genes are regulated by vitamin D_3, affecting everything from calcium metabolism to brain and muscle function to immunity. Vitamin D deficiency is now known to be a leading cause of the latitudinal differences in a variety of diseases.[10]

Natural sunlight is also necessary for the proper functioning of the pineal gland, which regulates the involuntary nervous system; it is therefore essential for maintaining the homeostasis (state of equilibrium) of every system in the body. In addition, during the winter months, when daylight is in short supply in the nontropical latitudes, many people begin to feel moody. In extreme cases of depression, this is called seasonal affective disorder and is treated with light therapy. If you have ever felt gloomy, low on energy, and irritable by mid-winter, now you know why.

Another reason that city life and man-made environments are so stressful is the gaping absence of true nature in them. Our ancestors were intimately aware of their biological connection to nature, but we are not. One of the most unfortunate aspects of the modern lifestyle is our physical, psychological, and spiritual loss of this profound relationship. Doesn't this make sense, considering that we emerged from nature?

From birth, being outdoors in nature should be part of our life-style. Unfortunately, children are spending more time indoors today than ever before, watching TV, playing video games, and using computers. Research has shown that outdoor playtime has declined by at least 50 percent since 1981.[11] School-age children spend an average of forty-four hours per week—more than six hours a day—in front of an electronic screen of one kind or another.[12]

This is unfortunate, because there is scientific evidence that child development is positively affected by contact with nature, especially wild nature. One study concluded that the key components of a child's psychological development—traits like self-esteem, self-confidence, self-concept, and autonomy—are enhanced by being in nature.[13] Other research has shown that natural environments reduce stress in children and facilitate learning.[14] Children with attention-deficit/hyperactivity disorder experience a reduction of their symptoms of distraction while playing in green settings.[15] And regularly being outside in a natural setting improves children's long-distance vision.[16]

None of these facts are surprising when you consider the underlying reasons. Our brains receive a continuous stream of information from the environment through electrochemical impulses that are triggered by our physical senses. Thus, our thoughts and moods are directly affected by our physical activity and location. Like an antenna, the body is exquisitely sensitive, continuously sensing the environment. Even without the involvement of the conscious mind, it is sending messages through the nervous system to the brain—which then instructs the cells on what kinds of hormones to release into the bloodstream—and is also picking up on subtle electromagnetic signals. Our bodies, minds, and spirits are always exchanging energy and information through a constant, dynamic stream of bi-directional feedback.

THE STRESS OF TECHNOLOGY

Repeated exposure on television to scenes of natural disasters (like hurricanes and earthquakes) and acts of violence (like the real events of 9/11 and school shootings or the fictional murders and rapes you see in dramas) can cause severe distress and even post-traumatic stress disorder in some viewers. If someone has had an actual experience of abuse or trauma, these images can cause anxiety and nightmares. If you sense yourself becoming disturbed and upset by something you see on television, you should limit your exposure. A basic rule for all of us is to watch the news once, if we want to be informed, and then turn it off.

Do you sit in front of a computer several hours a day? If so, you are not alone. But you should be mindful that 90 percent of people who spend more than three hours a day on computers experience blurred vision, eyestrain, and eye irritation. Repetitive strain disorder, as these symptoms are known, appears to be increasing by leaps and bounds.[17]

A behavioral study of 1,000 people that measured their awareness and short-term memory found that the pressures of modern life and our nonstop use of technology has cut our attention spans in half in less than a decade. Absence of attention puts us at risk for impairment of task performance and increases the likelihood of accidents in the home and while driving. It also interferes with our ability to remember simple daily events.[18]

The Institute of Psychiatry at the University of London suggests that technology is so distracting and disruptive that our IQ falls ten points when we're multitasking and dealing with constant e-mails, text messages, and phone calls. This is twice as bad as the decline in cognitive ability from smoking marijuana and comparable to the loss of cognitive ability from missing an entire night's sleep.[19]

SLEEP IS AN ENVIRONMENTAL ISSUE

How are you sleeping? Are you having challenges going to sleep or staying asleep, or are you waking up not revitalized? Sleep is the time your body and mind have the opportunity to regenerate and reinvigorate themselves. Having a good night's sleep on a regular basis is a key ingredient of superhealing. Unfortunately, and sometimes tragically, sleep is becoming an increasingly significant health issue throughout the modern world.

The long-term absence of a good night's sleep, defined as sleep that is not only restful but also restorative and revitalizing, is related to many growing health issues. The U.S. Centers for Disease Control estimate that between 50 and 70 million adults, almost half of the adult population, have experienced a sleep or wakefulness disorder (such as falling asleep unintentionally, dozing while driving, or having difficulty falling asleep).[20] Sleep deficiency is linked to automobile accidents, work-related errors, and industrial disasters because it causes memory impairment, difficulty in making decisions, loss of attention span, loss of memory, and reduced cognitive ability.[21]

It's hard to believe, but sadly and often tragically true, that very few people regularly get a good night's sleep anymore. Insomnia becomes more common later in life, especially among women, whereas men and obese people are more likely to develop a condition known as sleep apnea, in which breathing stops brieflyor becomes very shallow. Untreated sleep apnea contributes to the likelihood of the development of chronic diseases, including heart attack, stroke, and diabetes.[22]

Intrusive use of modern technology, such as television viewing in the bedroom and continual attention to computer screens and smartphones, is believed to be a factor in chronic sleep deprivation. Too much noise, light, and mental stimulation of any kind make it difficult to sleep. The cure for insomnia and interrupted sleep can include installing blackout curtains on your bedroom windows, wearing earplugs and an eye mask, and practicing good sleep hygiene. The National Sleep Foundation advises avoiding stimulants like coffee, nicotine, alcohol, and chocolate close to bedtime; getting vigorous exercise early in the day and doing relaxing exercise, such as yoga or tai chi, in the evening; establishing a regular relaxing bedtime routine; and making sure that both the bed and conditions in the bedroom are comfortable.[23]

THE PSYCHOLOGICAL BENEFITS OF NATURE

I've often heard people describe mountains as cathedrals and use other religious metaphors to describe the spiritual awe they feel in the presence of a majestic canyon or a waterfall. These comparisons are appropriate. Nature's wondrous design uplifts mind, body, and spirit. It causes our emotions to soar when we come in contact with it.

Although we know intuitively that being in touch with nature is healthy because it feels good and refreshing to be outdoors, now there's a convincing and growing body of research confirming that it contributes to mental health and psychological development. Nature benefits us by improving self-confidence and self-discipline, deepening our sense of community and belonging, and strengthening our sense of internal coherence.

We may have forgotten it, but our most distant ancestors knew they were connected to and part of the landscape. Since the human race evolved in the midst of nature, it is only logical that being in its presence is one of the fastest ways to align mind, body, and spirit and open our channels of superhealing. It helps us to remember. Like nothing else, experiencing nature consciously connects us to the magnificence of our true essence, our spirit. By engaging our sense of wonder, it leads us to feel appreciation for something greater than ourselves. It teaches us that although we are individuals, we are connected to a larger whole—to all of life. Its grandeur reminds us that there is something beyond what we, as human beings, could create, something timeless and unbound by the constraints of human intervention and involvement.

Nature affects us in a variety of positive ways, some of which are easily measured and some of which are not measurable but are meaningful and important nonetheless. Our exposure to a variety of colors, plants, mountains, forests, and seas, with their soothing sounds and fragrant odors, as well as the energy of different places, restores our sense of health and well-being. A 2010 study discovered that spending just twenty minutes outdoors in nature gave people a greater sense of well-being and vitality, beyond what is caused merely by having engaged in physical activity or enjoyable social interactions. Wilderness excursion participants reported that just remembering their outdoor experiences enhanced their health and happiness.[24]

Exposure to natural landscapes stimulates the parasympathetic nervous system, triggering the relaxation response and the release of endorphins. This reduces the stress hormones circulating in our bodies, lowers blood pressure, and helps to relieve anxiety, anger, aggression, and depression.[25] The opportunity to see nature, even through a window, accelerates recovery after surgery, shortening postoperative hospital stays.[26] Other studies have determined that prison rooms with a view of a natural landscape were beneficial to the health of prisoners.[27]

When we're in natural settings, we are known to recover more quickly from stress. Researchers at the University of Michigan (Ann Arbor) and Uppsala University (Sweden) have found that mental fatigue is relieved by nature experiences. Nature creates a sense of wonder and fascination that counterbalances the effects of too much focused attention, such as that required to use electronic devices like computers and smartphones. After an hour of taxing mental work, a walk through a park is more mentally and emotionally restorative than a walk through a city, reading a magazine or a book, or listening to music. The restorative effects of walking in nature trigger renewed attention and positive moods.[28]

In addition, nature improves our social relationships and our perceptions of other people. University of Rochester researchers found that after viewing scenes of nature, people were kinder and more compassionate and giving, as demonstrated by their willingness to donate money to a charity. The exposure also caused them to feel heightened concern about social outcomes and closer to members of their community. The researchers concluded that exposure to nature helps us get in touch with our basic values.[29]

Dwelling in nature can lead to more opportunities for physical activity, which keeps us fit and offers us relief from the demands of our daily lives.[30] More than 100 studies show that stress is decreased by participation in outdoor recreation.[31]

To activate your innate superhealing capabilities, it is imperative for you to design your lifestyle in such a way that you may take full advantage of the benefits of nature. Exposure to the natural environment is one of the most underutilized but powerful pathways to optimal health. Even if you live in an urban setting, it is important to be in contact with nature as much as possible. Add natural elements to your home, such as indoor plants, and allow fresh air and natural sunlight to come in through the windows. Make a point of visiting parks and recreational areas.

If you are fortunate to live in close proximity to nature, as my husband and I do, take advantage of the landscape around your home. Go outside and walk, bike, swim, climb, garden, and even sit where you can allow yourself the gift of nature's presence.

GARDENING AND HORTICULTURAL THERAPY

Before I went to medical school at Duke University, I didn't fully appreciate nature. That changed during my first winter in North Carolina, when I saw some of the most magnificent sunsets I've ever laid eyes on. These spectacles were so breathtaking that drivers would often pull off the road to watch them. I later learned that sand from the Sahara Desert is sometimes carried by the wind across the Atlantic Ocean to the North Carolina coastline, where it provides a canvas for the sun. Dramatic hues of red, pink, orange, and lavender looked like interlacing ribbons wrapping around the sun as it sank below the horizon.

Medical school and the exposure my training in medicine gave me to ill, injured, and dying patients was stressful. One day, after seeing a terminally ill patient, I didn't know what to do with my turbulent thoughts and feelings. I rushed out of the hospital and sat in the Sarah P. Duke Gardens, conveniently located behind the hospital, until I was able to recover my internal balance. My distress seemed to melt away. Created by the Duke family, this garden contains flowers and trees gathered from around the world. From that day forward, I had a favorite spot near a pond across from a terraced section filled with flowers. There I'd sit, inhaling the beauty—sometimes for hours, especially during the many weekends I was on call in the hospital.

My parents gardened. As a child, I spent a lot of time looking at my mother's flowers. But it wasn't until I planted my own garden outside the house where I now live that I came to appreciate how truly wondrous it is to watch a seed grow. It is amazing. Every summer,

I grow herbs, peppers, and tomatoes on my deck and flowers in the garden. I find putting my hands in the soil and tending my plants to be therapeutic.

According to the American Horticultural Therapy Association, the healing benefits of gardens has been recognized and incorporated into medical treatment since the time of the Egyptians. In Europe, 600 years ago, patients gardened with monks as part of their treatment. Dr. Benjamin Rush, a signer of the U.S. Declaration of Independence, astutely recognized the clinical improvement that people with mental illness experienced after participating in gardening. Gardening was widely used to help World War II veterans overcome the trauma of their experiences in battle. Some prisons have developed gardening programs for rehabilitative purposes, and placing healing gardens and spaces in hospitals and public settings is gaining momentum.[32]

EARTH ENERGY

As a child, I loved playing in mud. Did you? And oh, those mud pies! They were quite delicious to my adventurous palate, not that I now recommend them as an appetizer. What I never guessed is that having contact with soil for energetic reasons is a simple way to prevent illness and enhance healing. I enjoyed playing outside in the dirt, and in my adult years, walking along beaches during vacations is one of my most favorite activities. Now I understand why.

According to groundbreaking research, walking barefoot on soil or on grass connects us to Earth's natural electrical currents. Earthing, or grounding, as this technique is known, enables our feet to receive electrons, which enhances health by reducing inflammation (and the stress response) that is the biochemical foundation of numerous chronic disorders. Earthing also thins the blood, regulates our organs' natural rhythms, improves sleep, and reduces chronic pain.[33]

One of my favorite things to do is to walk barefoot on a beach. If you've ever enjoyed that experience or the sensations of walking barefoot in a grassy field, it is partly because you were in contact with the vitality of the planet itself. The transfer of energy from earthing causes an immediate sense of well-being and relaxation.

SUPERHEALING WORK SHEET: YOUR RELATIONSHIP WITH NATURE

1. What is your relationship with nature?
2. How often do you find yourself in nature's midst?
3. Are you taking advantage of the benefits of nature?
4. How often do you take a walk in a park or escape the city?
5. How often do you enjoy engaging with nature?
6. When was the last time you felt a moment of awe in the midst of nature?
7. Describe how that experience made you feel.
8. How would you like to enhance your experience with nature?
9. Can you add a little bit of nature to your home or office (plants, flowers, pictures)?
10. How have electronic devices, such as your computer and cell phone, affected your life?
11. Do you multitask?
12. Are you easily distracted?
13. Do you want to change your being easily distracted?

CHAPTER 5

SUPERHEALING WITH MOVEMENT

*"The real dance is a spontaneous body movement
that in harmony with the beats of the music in your heart."*

—*Toba Beta*

MY PARENTS TAUGHT ME A LOT ABOUT HEALTH. TWO OF THE HEALTH-iest people I've ever known, they were very active throughout their lives and had a love of life that was inspiring. Besides gardening, they exercised regularly—in fact, they did so many physical activities that I can't remember half of them. They were great role models. As a family, we spent a lot of time in our backyard, playing games, barbecuing, and working on the house.

One critical episode with my parents changed my life. For a gift, I had brought them to one of my favorite places in the world: Montego Bay, Jamaica. They were already in their early seventies and I was in my midthirties. It was a beautiful tropical day. The rays of the hot sun beat down on us as we strolled up a steep hill after spending a day at the beach. We were heading back toward the guesthouse where we were staying. Before the trip, I had worried that they would find it a challenge to walk up this hill, so for the first couple of days I sprang for a cab back from the beach. Then, to my surprise, they told me to save my money. They wanted to walk up the hill.

On this first trip by foot, we stopped halfway to rest on a shaded bench beneath a beautiful palm tree. After a few moments of chatting and catching our breath, my mother asked me, "Are you ready to go up?"

"No," I replied, still panting.

"Then see you at the top," she said. With that, she and my dad continued toward the house. After they'd gone, I remained on the bench for a few more minutes and watched them glide up the rest of the steep incline, seemingly effortlessly and with energy to spare. I realized how out of shape I was. *What's wrong with this picture?* I asked myself.

I am the first to admit that because of my busy schedule, I haven't always made exercise a priority or taken care of myself as well as I should. I'd known that I was out of condition and needed to exercise, but I'd been avoiding taking action. My parents' example lit a fire under me. As soon as I got home, I joined a local health club, and for the next ten years, I exercised there at least three days a week. I was much better for it.

But then I fell back into my old habits, and my exercise regimen slacked off. Part of my problem—or, I should say, my challenge—has been not only finding the time in my schedule for working out but also committing myself emotionally to doing it. Like many people, I have a love-hate relationship with exercise. I know it's good for me, and I enjoy it once I get going, but even so, I don't always do it. On some level, I equate exercising with flossing my teeth: it's got proven benefits and really should be done daily. Despite all my good intentions, however, I've often found it easy to put off exercising until "tomorrow."

Of course, I'm not alone. Recent surveys indicate that 75 percent of Americans don't get much exercise. This high degree of inactivity has a detrimental effect on the muscles, the internal organs, and the brain. In a multitude of ways it makes people more susceptible to a variety of chronic disorders, putting them at risk for heart disease, stroke, diabetes, and dementia when they get older. The adage "Use it or lose it" is very apt.

Older and wiser, I turned over a new leaf a few years ago. I began to pay more attention to my health and resumed my former gym regimen. As a result, I honestly feel better now than I have felt for years. This time around, I have made it a point to choose activities that I find fun. Thus I participate in a couple of dance-based fitness classes each week, and I'm having a ball. I can also actually feel my body thanking me for exercising. My mood is better. I'm losing weight (just in time for another high school class reunion), sleeping better, and feeling younger. These results are typical of what can be expected by anyone who engages in superhealing through physical activity.

In this chapter, we're going to discuss the dangers of a sedentary lifestyle and compare them to the positive effects of moderate and vigorous activity, which relieves stress, improves cardiovascular health, and retards the aging process, among other powerful outcomes. We'll also consider the benefits of movement in terms of the mind and the spirit and look at how we can involve the mind and our body awareness in activities that are otherwise primarily aimed at improving physical fitness. Vigorous, conscious movement is one of the most powerful components of the superhealing lifestyle.

Of course, other lifestyle factors are significant besides exercise: proper diet and hydration, moderate alcohol consumption, rest, and maintaining a positive attitude are also keys to superhealing. This does not mean you must change all of your unhealthy behavior patterns overnight, but it does mean you need to make a firm decision to begin changing them and then take steps that move you in the right direction.

THE DANGERS OF BEING SEDENTARY

Are you a couch potato, lying around watching TV for hours on end in the evenings and on the weekends? Do you spend many hours seated at a desk during the day? Thanks in part to the technology revolution, it's very likely that you do. If so, you should know that there is a relationship between long stretches of sitting and dying from heart disease. This risk to your health is heightened even if you do physical activity at other times.[1]

We are in the midst of an epidemic of chronic disease related to the modern lifestyle. The sedentary behavior now ingrained in our culture is literally killing us. Long periods sitting in front of a computer or driving a vehicle, such as a bus or a taxicab, have a significant negative effect on our physiology.[2] For example, extended TV viewing—the kind that's done while seated in your living room or lying down on a couch or in bed rather than while running on a treadmill at the gym—leads to an increased incidence of metabolic syndrome, a precursor of diabetes, in adults over sixty.[3]

The solutions can be simple. In my workplace, for example, I intentionally asked not to have a printer installed in my office so that I would have to get out of my chair routinely and walk ten feet or so over to the shared printer. I also make a point to stand up and stretch periodically, because I sit at my desk or in meetings for at least four or five hours every day. It is critical to interrupt your prolonged periods of sitting by standing up and walking around.[4] Other options would be to take phone calls standing up or to do your paperwork while standing at a high counter.

Researchers now believe that sedentary behavior should be considered the actual cause of the majority of human diseases. Being sedentary has been proved to increase the risk of heart disease by 45 percent, the risk of osteoporosis by 59 percent, the risk of stroke by 60 percent, and the risk of high blood pressure by 30 percent.[5] Although most people are clearly aware that exercise is essential, almost 75 percent of people don't achieve the necessary level of activity to prevent these illnesses.[6]

THE PHYSICAL BENEFITS OF MOVEMENT

If you're thinking about staying young at heart, fit, and strong as you grow older and want to engage your superhealing capacities, the best thing you can do is to get off the couch or step away from your computer or other favorite technological gadget and *move*. Many people now wear pedometers to measure the number of steps they are taking. Guidelines published by the federal government state the importance of walking 10,000 steps a day. But the intensity of your exercise also matters. When you do moderately intense activity or vigorous activity, your body will reward you.

The Centers for Disease Control define moderately intense exercise as activities like walking at a brisk pace of 100 steps per minute (3,000 steps per half hour), biking five to nine miles per hour on flat terrain, doing light calisthenics or yoga, golfing, ballroom dancing, playing doubles tennis, canoeing, playing Frisbee, and swimming recreationally. Vigorous activity is defined as activities like jogging or running five miles per hour or faster, biking more than ten miles per hour or on steep terrain, doing high-impact aerobics, jumping rope, wrestling or boxing, playing singles tennis, playing soccer or racquetball, and swimming steady laps.[7]

Moderate exercise is good for us. Exercising moderately for thirty minutes a day, five days a week, has been shown through projections and comparisons to population data, in terms of life expectancy, to lower rates of premature death by 19 percent in people who were previously inactive.[8] Vigorous exercise is even more beneficial. Fifteen to twenty minutes of vigorous activity every day produces improved cardiovascular function, reduced abdominal body fat, and lowered stress. Furthermore, studies have shown that short bursts of exercise, such as at ten-minute intervals, may be just as good for improving metabolic health and reducing the risk for chronic disease as longer durations of sustained exercise.[9]

Exercise is a characteristic of your lifestyle—entirely under your control—that will help you be healthier in ways you might not even imagine until you begin a regular fitness regimen. I've exercised most of my adult life—except for a few years, and especially since the vacation with my parents in Jamaica—and I can tell you that when I'm not exercising vigorously several times a week, I simply do not feel as good. When I don't move regularly, I feel both physically and mentally stagnant. When I am active, in contrast, I feel confident that nothing is impossible for me to accomplish.

If you are not aware that exercise is one of the most effective antiaging strategies available to you, it's probably because it requires more effort from us than the packaged creams, procedures, pills, surgeries, and everything else that's advertised to us as a means to appear younger. Study after study has shown, however, that exercise keeps our cells, organs, and bodies young. If exercise was a drug, it would probably be the bestselling drug ever, because it impedes the aging process, prevents the development of chronic disease, and, by virtue of the biochemicals and neural pathways it activates, relieves depression and anxiety and uplifts our moods.

One of the most important things exercise does is to protect our telomeres, the caps on the strands of our DNA, from the damage induced by stress, which makes it an important way to prevent aging. A study of women who were chronically stressed from taking care of a loved one with Alzheimer's disease showed that exercising protected their telomere length.[10] A study of middle-aged athletes showed that the telomeres in those who exercised were longer than the telomeres of those who didn't. The same researchers evaluated mice and found that those that ran for three weeks experienced increased levels of the protective proteins that maintain the length of telomeres and postpone the process of cell death.[11]

People approaching the sixth and seventh decades of their lives often become frightened and distressed about the prospect of losing their memories as they age and of developing Alzheimer's disease or another form of dementia. People in their forties and fifties, especially those with a family history of Alzheimer's, often worry, too. As a doctor, I'm frequently asked, "Is there anything I can do to prevent myself from developing Alzheimer's?" My answer is to reduce stress and begin a walking program.

EXERCISE AND MEMORY

Just a year of moderate exercise, such as walking, can increase the size of the hippocampus, which leads to improved memory. A study followed a group of nonexercising adults ages sixty to eighty who already were experiencing a natural shrinking of the hippocampus. When they began moderately intense walking, the improvements they experienced were the equivalent of turning back time two years. The researchers found that walking up to five miles a week protected the brain in people diagnosed with Alzheimer's and with mild cognitive impairment for a ten-year period.[12]

Performing moderate physical activity during midlife and late life appears to reduce mild cognitive impairment in people helping prevent the development of dementia, whereas a six-month high-intensity aerobic exercise program may improve cognitive function in individuals who already have dementia.[13] A moderate level of exercise during midlife has been associated with a 39 percent decrease in the likelihood of developing Alzheimer's.[14]

Cancer survivors often experience treatment-related health issues and a poorer quality of life. Exercise interventions are believed to help prevent these types of undesirable experiences, which are a particularly important factor in surviving cancer. A review of forty trials that evaluated 3,694 cancer patients (with cancers of the colon, breast, lymphatic system, head, and neck, among others) determined that exercise had a positive effect on their quality of life, compared to those who did not. They also experienced improvement of their body image, an enhanced sense of well-being, reduced fatigue and pain, and better sleep and social functioning.[15] A variety of activities was assessed, including strength training, walking, cycling, resistance training, yoga, tai chi, and qigong.

Physical activity has been known for many years to be an effective tool in the management of depression and other mood disorders, including anxiety and panic. All improve with regular engagement.[16]

What's beautiful is that it's never too late for anyone to begin to exercise, not even those approaching 100 years of age.[17] It's wise to start out gradually and build up the intensity and the duration. If you're a relatively sedentary person or someone over the age of fifty, you should discuss your exercise plan with your physician before beginning a new fitness regimen. Once you get the go-ahead, I'm sure you'll find that setting up a routine gives you momentum so that it becomes easier, and as a result you will feel better and younger.

EXERCISING WITH AWARENESS

An interesting study was conducted to determine what role, if any, the mind plays in receiving the health benefits of exercise. To investigate whether perception can improve a person's physical condition independently of actual exercise, the researchers compared two groups of hotel maids. The women's fitness levels were measured at the beginning of the study, and all were in poor health and considered themselves sedentary. None exercised regularly, two-thirds did so occasionally, and the rest didn't exercise at all. More than half were told something they did not know: that cleaning fifteen rooms a day involves more physical activity than is required to meet the U.S. surgeon general's recommendation of thirty minutes of daily physical activity. They were also given details about the number of calories their activities burned. The others, those making up the control group, were not informed of these things.[18]

Four weeks later, the health status of the hotel maids was reevaluated. Those in the group that had been informed had lost an average of two pounds and experienced a 10 percent reduction in their blood pressure. They were significantly healthier, as determined by body fat percentage, body mass index, and waist-to-hip ratio, than the maids who were not informed of caloric expenditures and daily exercise guidelines. The health changes they had undergone were especially remarkable because they occurred so quickly and were much higher than those experienced by the uninformed control group. On some level, the simple act of explaining that what forty-four hotel maids were doing each day was significant exercise was sufficient to improve their health substantially.[19]

This is a pretty amazing finding, in my opinion, and it complements other studies that have found that athletes benefit from the visualization they do of participating in their sports. Through brain activation by imagery, their muscles are stimulated as though they are physically engaged in the sport.[20] Before the U.S. Olympic trials and the Olympic Games in Seoul, South Korea, in 1988, track and field athletes found that preevent visualization improved their performance.[21] A study involving elite gymnasts found that those who made the Olympic team had ways of thinking, affirming, and visualizing success that could be strongly linked to superior gymnastic performance. Affirmations and certain forms of mental imagery seemed to differentiate the best gymnasts from the gymnasts who failed to make the Olympic team. These two types of gymnasts also appeared to show different anxiety patterns and different methods of coping with competitive stress.[22]

Do you pay attention to what you're doing? It's easy for the mind to wander off so that we become unaware of what's going on in our bodies. If you are usually only partly aware of what you're doing, especially when you're exercising, remind yourself that your perception can expand the benefits. Paying attention and engaging in simple positive self-talk can lead to the increased effectiveness of any fitness regimen.

Our minds have a remarkable capacity to change our physiology when we engage our bodies with awareness. This awareness has the capacity to affect every aspect of our daily lives. That mental imagery affects motor skill learning and performance has been known since the 1930s, and an analysis of sixty studies indicated that mental practice improves performance on cognitive tasks even more than on motor or strength tasks.[23]

A core component of superhealing movement is body awareness. For several reasons, paying attention to your body is a key ingredient of superhealing. As I often tell my patients, if you don't pay attention to its signals, your body first whispers, then it speaks, screams, slaps, and finally stops you—usually with an illness. That's why it is essential to respect its messages as early as possible. Responding to the body is something our society doesn't encourage us to do. In fact, we're often encouraged, and sometimes even required, to deny the natural impulses and messages of our bodies. But we do so at our own peril.

In particular, I'm thinking about the dangers of ignoring the stressful messages we receive. Of course, we can't pay attention to every twinge and discomfort we get during the day, but when we see a trend of disharmony occurring, we need to listen more closely. In our culture, we need to pay more attention to the body, to honor it with loving awareness, which is really one of the simplest and easiest things to do.

Many mind-body movement systems, including yoga, tai chi, and qigong, recognize awareness as a core mechanism of action. For therapeutic effect, these approaches usually combine intentional focus with breathing and movement. Practitioners of these systems understand that body awareness plays a role in the unfolding of greater self-awareness and the unity of body, mind, and spirit.[24]

Yoga, which is the Sanskrit word for "union," is an ancient mind-body-spirit healing path from India and Tibet. Although most Westerners associate yoga with physical postures, it is actually a collection of traditions related to, among other things, sound, breath, and movement. There are also yoga practices of action, devotion, and intellect. The movement techniques of yoga strengthen and increase the flexibility of the physical body, reduce stress, and promote well-being in a unique way: the postures engage the mind and spirit in the moment, which results in a biological shift that invokes the relaxation response by stimulating the parasympathetic nervous system.[25]

Yoga reduces stress, and in the process it decreases the levels of chemicals involved in chronic inflammation. This is not only an immediate experience that occurs while doing yoga. Yoga also regularly increases the practitioner's ability to respond to stressful encounters in such a way that an inflammatory response does not occur in the first place.[26]

A recent study investigated yoga's ability to correct an irregular heartbeat, known as atrial fibrillation. This serious, potentially life-threatening condition can be caused by work-related or emotional stress as well as by certain nutrient deficiencies. It occurs when the heart's natural electrical signals are triggered to fire off in a disorganized manner, causing the heart to quiver. When it becomes a disorder, it requires drug therapy or sometimes invasive treatment. Researchers found that people with chronic atrial fibrillation who did yoga experienced "significantly reduced" irregular heartbeat episodes compared to a control group that did other forms of exercise. The experimental group participants also reported lower levels of depression and anxiety, and their general health and vitality improved.[27]

Tai chi and qigong, which originated in the ancient Far East, are practices that, along with yoga, are considered a form of exercise known as meditative movement. These traditions share a common philosophy related to the movement of life-force energy, or chi, and similar patterns of movements.[28]

Between 1993 and 2007, seventy-seven published reports compared tai chi and qigong to other forms of exercise or to a sedentary lifestyle. A recent review of these studies involving more than 6,400 participants found that tai chi and qigong improved not only the practitioners' quality of life but also their hearts, lungs, and immune systems. Tai chi and qigong improved physical function, raised the quality of life, prevented falls, and enhanced the sense of self-worth and psychological health. Researchers believe that the combination of awareness, posture, and movement in these systems promotes a state of self-awareness that is more efficient than the normal state of awareness. This activates the release of beneficial chemicals throughout the body that promote self-healing.[29]

Apparently, the physiological and psychological changes induced by meditative movement profoundly enhance the body's regenerative and regulatory mechanisms on multiple levels. So keep in mind that a combination of physical exercise, meditation, and proper diet is a very effective way to trigger your capacity for superhealing.

THE SPIRITUAL BENEFITS OF MOVEMENT

Exercising is critical for optimal wellness, but it is only one part of the equation. Although exercise of any kind can help you release tension and manage stress, moving in a way that engages your spirit makes the biggest difference. When I first became health-conscious, I approached my body as though it were a machine that had fallen into disrepair. Spiritual engagement was reserved for Sunday morning church services. What I wasn't taking into consideration was the unimaginably powerful intelligence of Spirit, which I believe is the source that animates my being. I didn't know yet that I could tap into this intelligence, which lies at the heart of creation and represents life itself.

The common thread that links every chapter in this book, even this one on movement, is awareness. Much too often, we don't pay attention to our bodies, or if we do pay attention, it's in a way that's not in alignment with the true source of our wellness and healing. The human body is worth marveling at. It is an amazing organism, not at all like a machine. When we consciously engage in movement, wonderful things happen. Everything shifts. Our awareness gives us the capacity to heal. Conscious exercise has been found to help people cope better and survive longer even when they have the most serious and life-threatening diseases.

Our bodies are not designed not for stagnation but for movement. Nevertheless, isn't it interesting that people who meditate are usually seated and still? Their state is regenerative and restorative, so obviously they are in a different state of being from your run-of-the-mill television viewer or sedentary desk worker. Perhaps the issue with being seated, then, isn't so much the lack of movement as it is the lack of true stillness.

When we are simultaneously physically engaged and spiritually

engaged, we are aligned with the true source of our being and building our health. Physical activity is protective of our health, and so is
spiritual activity. Think of the Tibetan Buddhist monks who meditate
for hours on end to reach a state of *samadhi,* or union with the divine.
They can be buried alive for hours, deprived of normal amounts of
oxygen, and emerge unharmed. Think of the joggers who experience
a rush of endorphins, the brain's natural opiates or painkillers, and
report feeling high. Put the two activities together, and you have a real
opportunity for superhealing. What does a jogger have in common
with a monk? An opportunity for an awakening of epic proportions.

Although brain function may, to a certain extent, determine what
a runner and a meditator have in common, I believe there is a higher
energy or intelligence involved in the meditator's activity that cannot be fully or adequately measured at this time. Meditation engages
the brain in a way that is highly beneficial to us. The brain-wave and
chemical patterns related to our normal waking behavior do not.

Perhaps the true danger of the sedentary lifestyle is not the inactivity per se but rather the lack of conscious engagement with
our spirit when we're "vegging out." Our culture's typical absence of
awareness and our preoccupation with tuning out with computers
and TV as a form of emotional coping may be unconscious sources
of stress that are harming our bodies. Perhaps we should tune in
to our spirits instead. This is just a hunch, but I believe it is a good
one—and worth pursuing. Physical inactivity, as we know it, with
its attending risk factors for disease, may not be harmful primarily
because of the inactivity, but rather because of the disruption of our
spiritual activity and body awareness.

When you're engaged in movement that brings you peace and joy,
you can gain access to the higher pathways your being that allow the
high energy of spirit to clearly flow through you.

SUPERHEALING WORK SHEET: ASSESSING YOUR PHYSICAL ENGAGEMENT

Are you ready to move, or engage your body and being physically, with ever-increasing awareness? It's never too late to begin. Even exercising during an illness is helpful, but rarely are we encouraged to do so. Ask yourself the following questions:

- How much activity are you doing now?
- What sort of exercise are you doing?
- What are you doing that you enjoy?
- Are you getting a sufficient amount of exercise?
- Are you motivated to exercise?
- What physical activity are you willing to do?
- What attention do you give to your body?
- Do you listen to your body or ignore it?
- How do you feel about it?
- What are your thoughts about it?
- Do you heed the initial voice of distress, the whispers of fear, the call for rest, and the need for relaxation?
- Do you compliment your body or focus on what you think is flawed?
- How are you treating your body?
- How do you honor your body?

CHAPTER 6

SUPERHEALING WITH NUTRITION

"Let food be your medicine and medicine be your food."

—*Hippocrates*

WHEN I FIRST BECAME HEALTH-CONSCIOUS DURING MY TWENTIES, I FO-
cused on using food—among other things—to create physical
health. But I shortchanged myself, because I did not give any serious
thought to the effect that stress or my emotions had on my digestive
system. It took me many years of practicing better eating habits and
mindfulness to develop a greater awareness and appreciation of what
really matters about food and nutrition.

When I first began to focus on my health, I believed that eating a
plant-based diet and exercise alone would be my path to wellness. I
had never been a big meat eater, so this decision was aligned with my
personal preferences. Even today I don't eat animal protein, with the
rare exception of seafood. Over time, I discovered that I needed to
supplement my largely vegetarian diet with vitamins, minerals, fish
oil, and probiotics. I also needed to pay close attention to my stress
level and practice mindfulness when I ate. My route to superhealing
and optimal wellness has had many features.

I find it interesting that there is conflicting information on the biological necessity of limiting consumption exclusively to plant-based
foods, or even, as some people believe, to raw fruits and vegetables.
If you think you must eat meat, it's important to do your best to eat
meat from free-ranging, happy animals that were not raised on antibiotics or growth hormones, because those are the only kind that are

healthy for our bodies to ingest. Many people choose to be vegetarian for ethical reasons, which is a different matter entirely from the concern over the nutritive content of specific ingredients. I would never advise someone who disapproves of the way a particular food arrives on the table to eat that food, because its inclusion in the diet could trigger a nocebo effect (the negative influence one can experience just from believing something is harmful). How we feel about what we eat affects our physical responses to that food.

Even though vegetarianism has much to commend it, some people feel deprived after eliminating meat or another ingredient from their diets. Missing a food that they like to eat or that is familiar to them causes them to become stressed and feel sad. Some people's bodies fare better when fish and lean meats are included in their diets. Every individual has to determine what he or she needs, using, to some extent, trial and error.

I've learned that some especially resilient people can routinely eat pretty much whatever they want to eat—including meat and all kinds of things that are not considered good for us, like sugary treats and salty potato chips—yet they do not develop the predictable illnesses that come from consuming meat and refined foods. My observations have taught me that our bodies have a remarkable capacity to adapt to our diets if we're not operating in a crisis mode caused by stress and environmental challenges.

That being said, the latest scientific research proves the power of a largely plant-based diet rich in phytonutrients (*phyto* means "plant") to prevent and even reverse chronic disease. There is evidence that we benefit immensely from the regular consumption of raw fruits and vegetables; these are filled with enzymes that aid digestion, antioxidants that protect us from cellular degradation, and biophotons, the life force that originates from sunlight. These are the cornerstones of a superhealing nutritional plan that is appropriate for everyone. Today, those of us who live in developed nations have more food choices than ever before, yet we are increasingly unhealthy because of our excessive consumption of highly processed foods, which are lacking in vital nutrients.

Does this mean we should be inflexible about our diets, never letting a morsel of dessert, a cooked entrée, or any type of "bad" food pass our lips? Throughout the years, I've discovered that we can overdo it when we're focusing on the purity of our food—and for some of us, this can even become a psychological disorder. I've met people who refuse to eat anything that they themselves haven't prepared, and they exhibit the fervor of zealots. Yet their strict avoidance of certain ingredients they disapprove of does not necessarily make them healthier. When people are obsessed with food, it doesn't make them happier, either, because their minds are bound up with constant thoughts of food.

When choosing what to eat, there is a middle ground between restriction and permissiveness that is a more balanced and healthier approach to nourishment. For superhealing to occur, for the ongoing maintenance of your health, and to provide your body with the nutrients it needs to function optimally on a cellular level, you must learn to recognize and address the mental and emotional factors in your life that inform your eating habits and find a way to eat that makes you healthy and happy.

In this chapter, we're going to discuss principles of healthy eating based on the most advanced science on how to optimize digestion and absorption, as well as the effect of food on our mental and emotional well-being. We'll look at what to include in your diet and what to exclude, keeping in mind the attitudes of mindfulness, inner peace, love, and gratitude. Since everything related to nutrition ultimately comes back to digestion, we'll start by taking a look at ways to support and improve that function.

THE GUT-MIND CONNECTION

Your gastrointestinal (GI) tract, or gut—terms for the stomach and intestines in combination—plays an important role in your health. The stomach is where food is broken down by digestion into the different nutritional components your body needs to function optimally: the macronutrients of protein, carbohydrates, fats, and fluids; and the micronutrients of vitamins, minerals, and phytochemicals. After food is digested, the intestines are where nutrient absorption occurs.

If we're lacking the acids and enzymes that aid in the digestion of specific types of nutrients, then foods such as milk, beans, onions, wheat, or fat (to name just a few possibilities) cannot be properly digested, absorbed, and assimilated. In that case, they can give us pain, flatulence, constipation, or diarrhea. Because we are individuals, not everyone is challenged by the same foods. Some of us aren't challenged at all.

It's easy to think of nutrition entirely as a matter of how well your body responds to the foods you eat. But food can affect your moods and thought processes, too, in either a positive or a harmful manner. Your mind and spirit will be adversely affected if for any reason you become malnourished. This means getting inadequate nutrition because you're not eating enough foods or the right foods or because you're failing to properly digest and absorb nutrients. The bidirectional communication between your body and your mind, and your body and your spirit, is a key reason for this.

Furthermore, emotional distress and negative thinking affect the digestive system. Many of us worry about our caloric intake and fear possible weight gain, yet we think less about the "ingredient" of our emotions and how they affect the GI tract's ability to properly digest and absorb food. An old adage advises, "Never eat when you're angry or with an enemy." Doing so causes physiological distress, which affects our digestive processes. Eating while happy, relaxed, and content allows for appropriate absorption and assimilation of the nutrients in our food. Eating while stressed, in contrast, leads to indigestion.

Stress causes the release of cortisol and other hormones that alter digestion, causing changes in blood flow to the intestinal tract and increasing the flow of digestive acids. Excess acid can impair the production of enzymes released by your liver and pancreas and impede the flow of bile from the liver, which is essential for the digestion of fats. Stress hormones also influence muscle tone and tension. They can trigger muscular contractions throughout the body, including in the diaphragm, which is involved in breathing; in the muscles involved in swallowing; and in peristalsis, that moves food through the stomach and the large and small intestines. For these reasons, digestion is affected not only by what you eat but also by how you're feeling when you're eating and by what's already present in your intestinal tract.

In the worst-case scenario, stress can be so severe that it leads to the fight-or-flight response and entirely shuts down digestion so your body can use its energy elsewhere.

There are an extraordinary number of nerve cells in the gastrointestinal tract, leads many to call it the peripheral brain. To activate your superhealing capabilities, you need to become fully aware of what this "brain" is telling you and learn to honor the gut-mind connection. Your sense of well-being (or lack of it) plays a significant role in digestion, absorption, and immunity, which are three of the pillars of physical health.

We are all aware of the unpleasant gut feelings that we can get at times, such as nervous butterflies or the sensation of heartburn that we get when we're feeling stressed. The common symptoms of anxiety and depression involve the gut. In 1833, Dr. William Beaumont became the first to report on this phenomenon. He found that upsetting emotions decrease the secretion of stomach acids and prolong the emptying of the stomach after eating. He made these observations while treating a man with a fistula, or an external opening, caused by an accidental gunshot injury.[1]

Several physiologists conducting research on dogs subsequently identified that the vagus nerve, which extends from the brain stem down through the organs located in the neck and chest to the gastrointestinal organs in the abdomen, is required for normal interactions between the gut and the brain to occur.[2]

In fact, we now know that the intestinal tract contains more nerve cells than the entire rest of the body does; the number is second only to the number of nerve cells in the brain.[3]

Your GI tract's nervous system also sends sensory information to your brain that affects your emotional state, your memory, and other functions of thinking, including decision making. It produces 95 percent of the serotonin in your body, as well as other neurotransmitters once thought to exist exclusively in the central nervous system.[4]

Serotonin is a critical neurotransmitter that influences our sense of well-being and is a key mediator of the relationship between the gut and the brain. Low levels of serotonin have been implicated in a variety of psychiatric disorders, from depression and attention deficit disorder to anxiety and post-traumatic stress disorder.[5] Folate, a form of vitamin B that is found in leafy green vegetables (like spinach, broccoli, and lettuce), and protein foods that contain the amino acid tryptophan (like poultry, fish, eggs, nuts, and beans) boost the serotonin level, and so does the proper digestion and absorption of these foods.[6]

Certain foods have chemical properties that can make us more resilient against stress. We have all had the experience, for instance, of eating a favorite comfort food in response to a distressing experience and feeling better afterward. Generally, foods that give us emotional relief contain large amounts of fat. To study this phenomenon, Belgian researchers enlisted the participation of twelve healthy people to determine whether the consumption of fat actually changes the way the brain functions when we're sad. The participants were given either salt water or a liquid fat solution through a feeding tube. Then they listened to music characterized as emotionally neutral or sad while looking at matching images of neutral or sad faces, and they were asked to rate their moods and their sense of fullness or hunger several times. Those who received the fat solution felt approximately 50 percent less sadness compared to those who received the salt water.[7]

Consciously choosing your foods for nutritional value and the satisfaction they give you and consciously engaging in the act of eating are the foundation of physical health. Nutrition is not just what you eat; it's a lot more than that. You receive more or less nutritional value from the same foods depending on your perception of your food and how you're feeling at the time you're eating. If you're stressed, angry, or unhappy, your gut will digest quite differently than it does when you feel happy, joyful, or at peace.

EATING WITH AWARENESS
AND JOYFUL APPRECIATION

Do you eat your meals in the awareness of the present moment, paying close attention to your food, or are you distracted, even multitasking, while eating? There is good evidence that mindful eating improves our satisfaction and our satiation. When nutrients are absorbed, hormones are released that send signals to the brain of a sense of fullness and nonhunger that lasts long after a meal is over.[8]

Eating with gratitude and in pleasant surroundings improves the way your body digests and absorbs food. Eating while in a negative state of being or in an unpleasant environment is more challenging and taxing. Therefore, it's important to prepare yourself emotionally for your meals. If you're stressed, sad, tired, despairing, or angry, take a few moments before you eat to alter your mental and emotional state of being. If you're feeling any type of distress, it is imperative to take a few deep breaths, relax, and center yourself. Consciously shift your attention to a higher thought about an issue that's troubling you, or deliberately choose to think about something else.

Then, since nutrition is a matter not only of what you eat but of how you're feeling while you're eating, it is important to eat with awareness, slowly savoring each mouthful. Eat with attention, clarity, and awareness.

SUPERHEALING RECOMMENDATIONS
FOR MINDFUL EATING

I highly recommend the following principles for eating:

Take one or a few deep breaths and give thanks for your food before eating. Bless all who touched the food, from seed planter to meal preparer.

- If you're cooking, cook with love. There's nothing more scrumptious than a home-cooked meal made with love as a main ingredient.
- Eat when you're happy. Don't eat when you're sad or upset in any way, if you can avoid it.
- Pay attention to every morsel of your meal. Be present and savor it.

- Minimize distractions. Do not eat in your car, while watching TV, or while using your computer or phone.
- Slow down, chew thoroughly, and enjoy eating.

MAINTAINING YOUR COMMUNITY OF INTESTINAL FLORA

I had taken a short course of antibiotics to resolve a case of bronchitis I couldn't shake. I knew my illness could be attributed to sheer exhaustion, since I'd been working two jobs for more than fourteen months and my body was reeling from my failure to take better care of it. The combination of overwork and not enough sleep had taken its toll on me physically, emotionally, and spiritually, and something was wrong.

One day, about a month later, I ate a small slice of delicious fruitcake soaked in Jamaican rum. About an hour or so later, I began to feel a very gentle gnawing in the middle of my lower abdomen. Soon it felt like my intestines were going to rupture. The gas in my gut was expansive and felt like a balloon stretched to its limit. It was the most unbearable pain of my life.

Months later, after several on-again, off-again bouts of the same severe abdominal pain, I was really sick. I did everything I knew to alleviate my condition, but every natural therapy I tried caused the severe abdominal pain to return with a vengeance. Nearly a year after it had started, what began as a monthly bout of severe abdominal pain and distress ultimately engulfed the entire month, during which I writhed on the floor in pain. I couldn't do anything but moan.

It turned out that I'd developed irritable bowel syndrome from a yeast overgrowth triggered by the antibiotics. It wasn't until I learned how to rebalance my gut flora that I successfully recovered. Once I had my diagnosis in hand, I cleaned up my diet: I entirely avoided ingredients known to nourish yeast, and I supplemented what I ate with probiotics, the bacteria that maintain the healthy balance of microorganisms in the gut, such as the *Lactobacillus acidophilus* found in yogurt and fermented food.

Did you know that the number of bacterial cells living in your GI tract is estimated to be ten times more (over 100 trillion) than the entire number of number of cells in the rest of your body? An important and remarkable aspect of the GI tract is the dynamic nature of the diverse bacteria and other organisms, known as intestinal flora, dwelling within it. The average GI tract contains 500 to 1,000 different species of bacteria. These microbial life forms residing in the gut make it the most complex environment that exists in your body.[9]

An analysis of the DNA in the GI tract found that it contains 3.3 million genes from the microorganisms living there, which is a vast number compared to the 23,000 genes present in the cells in the rest of the human body.[10] You're going to hear much more about this topic in the future, so I want to give you the inside track on this area of emerging scientific knowledge. Our understanding of the importance of keeping the community of microorganisms in the gut in balance is rapidly expanding.

Some intestinal flora is damaging to our health, such as the infectious bacteria *Streptococcus* (strep), *Staphylococcus* (staph), *Salmonella*, *Clostridium botulinum*, *E. coli*, and *Candida albicans* yeast. However, the vast majority of gut flora is believed to play a positive role in maintaining our health. It is symbiotic with us, providing us with several crucial, life-sustaining benefits, including the production of vitamins, protection from infection by destructive microorganisms, refinement of the immune system's response, and the ability of the cells lining the GI tract to mature.[11]

Gut health is an important aspect of the immune system, where invading microorganisms (like dangerous bacteria, yeasts, fungi, and viruses) are destroyed. If the population of microorganisms that live in your gut becomes unbalanced, or your immune response is underactive, you will respond as though you were being poisoned, and your health can really suffer. That's what a dramatic change in my intestinal flora did to me.

Disruption of the balance of intestinal flora can lead to the development of several chronic diseases, including inflammatory bowel disease, diabetes, metabolic syndrome, obesity, autoimmune disorders, arthritis, colon cancer, irritable bowel syndrome, autoimmune liver diseases, malnutrition, allergies, and autism. People with these conditions have been found to have communities of gut bacteria that are significantly different from those of healthy people.[12]

A healthy balance of microflora in the gut requires a greater number of health-promoting microorganisms, or probiotics, than disease-causing ones. The community of intestinal flora is affected by diet, genetic makeup, age, sex, and—what I discovered for myself a few years ago—level of stress.

As hard as it might be to believe, as part of the two-way communication system between your body and mind, your intestinal flora affects your emotional state. Research has revealed that particular probiotic strains can reduce the level of gastrointestinal symptoms caused by stress. As a result of emerging evidence that gut flora affects how well the brain and the spinal cord function, a group of researchers sought to determine whether taking probiotics could actually reduce emotional distress. For a month, the study participants were assessed on a daily basis for stress, anxiety, depression, anger, and hostility. The levels of stress hormones in their urine were monitored, and at the end of the study they were found to be much lower.[13]

Reestablishing normal intestinal flora in a gut that has become unbalanced may be challenging, but introducing healthy intestinal bacteria has resulted in very promising results in studies like this one. Taking probiotics every day has been shown to alleviate distress, pain, depression, anger, hostility, and anxiety in studies demonstrating beneficial psychological effects in healthy human volunteers.[14]

We know that inflammation in your intestinal tract affects your entire body, especially the brain. Chronic gastrointestinal inflammation creates anxious behavior because of the damaging chemical changes it triggers in the central nervous system that induce the release of stress hormones.[15] The most significant cause of inflammation in the body may occur within the intestinal tract, and the release of the chemicals involved in the process probably affects the brain as well as other organs and blood vessels. Inflammation is believed to play an important role in the development of depression, which frequently occurs in conjunction with heart disease, cancer, type 2 diabetes, and autoimmune and neurodegenerative diseases.

A growing number of clinical trials have demonstrated the positive effect of probiotics on suppressing the inflammatory process in the intestinal tract and in the brain, when they are taken in conjunction with fatty acids and vitamins D and B. Together these may improve the effectiveness of treating depression.[16]

Given that you are in good gut health—or working toward it—and practicing mindful, happy eating, what should be on the menu to activate superhealing? Let's take a look.

THE SUPERHEALING POWER
OF FRESH FRUITS AND VEGETABLES

One of my earliest nutrition teachers was Dr. Max Gerson, who learned to treat cancer successfully with an entirely nutritional, rather than pharmaceutical, approach, beginning in the late 1920s. His approach to treating a wide range of diseases was based on his belief that there was healing power in vegetables and fruits. His patients consumed large volumes of fresh vegetable juice and ate plant-based meals to give their bodies high levels of nutrients to regenerate themselves. Remarkable recoveries occurred.[17]

Although Dr. Gerson could not have known back then what the most recent scientific evidence shows, he was clearly on the trail of something important. We now know that fruits and vegetables are packed with essential nutrients, called phytochemicals, and with biophotonic (from sunlight) energy. All the evidence shows that a high daily intake of these foods promotes health.

There are many associations between the amount of fruits and vegetables consumed and the rate of developing chronic disease. The more fresh produce you eat, the more protection your body has from the prospect of their development. One of the most interesting studies I've recently read found that people who eat at least seven servings of fresh fruits and vegetables a day experience much less psychological distress than those who don't. Why wouldn't you eat seven servings of fruits and vegetables if they improved not only your physical health but also your emotional well-being?

Diet has been largely ignored by the researchers who are scientifically investigating the causes of happiness; still, some research has taken place that proves the foods we consume do play a role in our well-being. In a joint study conducted by researchers from Dartmouth College in New Hampshire and the University of Warwick in Britain, the eating habits of more than 80,000 people in England, Scotland, and Ireland were evaluated. The investigators found that happiness and well-being increased with the amount of vegetables and fruits eaten every day and that well-being peaked among those who consumed seven servings a day. A serving was defined as 2.8 ounces. Although most government health departments recommend eating five servings a day of fruits and vegetables to promote physical health and prevent cancer and heart disease, additional servings are necessary to support emotional well-being.[18]

Our mothers were right: Fruits and vegetables are the key to good health. The power of fresh fruits and vegetables to sustain and heighten our health and well-being cannot be overstated. Former President George H.W. Bush publicly acknowledged his dislike of broccoli and banned it from the menu on Air Force One and at the White House. Personally, I don't care for brussels sprouts, but there are so many other vegetables to choose from that taste doesn't have to be an issue.

Why are fresh fruits and vegetables so important? Although it may sound boring to some, it was quite exciting to me to learn that some of the most powerful chemicals known to science exist in produce and were not created in a laboratory to be drugs. The phytochemicals in fruits and vegetables have health benefits, including the prevention of cancer, heart disease, and inflammatory, neurological, and metabolic disorders. Phytochemicals offer great promise in preventing cancer and healing damaged brains, hearts, lungs, kidneys, and other organs. They have remarkable properties, including being anti-inflammatory, antioxidant, and anticarcinogenic; they also affect genes linked to cellular metabolism, prevent stress, aid in detoxification, and lower total and LDL cholesterol levels.[19]

Leading cancer research institutions are now exploring the power of phytochemicals not only to prevent but also to halt the growth of tumors. Studies have found that the positive effect of food on preventing several different types of cancer is caused by phytochemicals. It is a major area of current cancer treatment research, since phytochemicals play a major role in altering several steps in the development of cancer. Because of epigenetic changes, some phytochemicals apparently have the capacity to even cure some cancers.[20] Mother Nature's pharmacy is magnificent; and it's something a drug company could never have created in a million years!

Consume organic fruits and vegetables if you can afford them. My personal belief is that organic produce—that is, produce grown without the use of pesticides—provides greater nutritional value than nonorganic produce. And even if that isn't the case, as some farmers, scientists, and policy makers would argue, it is nonetheless best to lower your exposure to pesticides. Pesticides have been linked conclusively to the development of cancer and neurological disorders, such as Parkinson's disease, in humans.[21]

In addition to eating organic raw fruits and vegetables, I choose not to buy a lot of processed and packaged foods, even those made with organic ingredients, for one important reason: Some of them are laced with unhealthy chemicals, with flavor enhancers such as monosodium glutamate (MSG), and with soy by-products (such as textured vegetable protein, soy protein isolates, and soy oil). These chemicals trigger detrimental responses in your body that contribute to the development of a variety of diseases.

MSG is an amino acid (glutamate) that stimulates brain cells. It is known as an excitotoxin because its stimulation is so severe that the cells in certain areas of the brain die. This chemical has been linked to the development of several neurological disorders, including attention deficit disorder, Alzheimer's, and Parkinson's disease.[22] Soy and its by-products are unhealthy because they contain several different types of chemicals that interfere with the functioning of many organs and the absorption of certain nutrients.[23]

I'm like everyone else—I sometimes find myself picking up a bag of chips from a vending machine or a sandwich from a fast-food joint. However, many years ago, while contemplating food, I came to see the importance of eating food that comes from the earth as much as possible and to eliminate the rest. I've done my best to adhere to this notion, because it is clear that fresh fruits and vegetables do a superior job of nourishing my body, mind, and spirit.

Superhealing nutrition is about the energetic quality of food as much as it's about the nutrient value. Everything we eat originally draws energy from the sun. Through the process of photosynthesis, plants capture sunlight and convert some of it into particles known as biophotons. All living organisms—plants and the animals that consume them—store biophotons in the DNA of their cells. Biophotons are a coherent form of light that releases energy in the human body. We need this vital energy. Biophotons contain important information that helps to direct and regulate our cellular functions.[24]

The amount of biophotons present in a fruit or a vegetable is believed to indicate its nutritional status: the more biophotons present, the healthier the food. For this important reason, the healthiest way to consume a fruit or a vegetable is in its natural, raw, and freshest state.[25]

SUPERHEALING RECOMMENDATION: FOODS TO INCLUDE IN YOUR DIET

To create a balanced, healthy diet, eat a variety of foods and be sure to include those from the following lists. All have proven health benefits, to various degrees, including the prevention of chronic diseases like cancer, heart disease, hypertension, diabetes, and emphysema.

Foods from the Earth

- Leafy green vegetables: kale, spinach, collard greens, mustard greens, turnip greens, and chard

- Cruciferous vegetables: brussels sprouts, cabbage, cauliflower, and broccoli
- Berries: blueberries, strawberries, blackberries, raspberries, and goji berries
- Fruits: cherries, apples, grapes, oranges, lemons, limes, grapefruit, kiwi, mangoes, and bananas
- Root vegetables: onions, garlic, shallots, beets, carrots, and turnips, yams,
- Mushrooms: shiitake, reishi, maitake, portobello, button, and others
- Beans: lentils, kidney beans, pinto beans, navy beans, red beans, and black beans
- Nuts: walnuts, almonds, pecans, cashews, and macadamia nuts
- Seeds: sunflower seeds, hemp seeds, chia seeds, pumpkin seeds, and flaxseed
- Avocados
- Healthy vegetable oils: grape seed, olive, and walnut
- Teas: green, white, black, and rooibos
- Juices: freshly made from spinach, kale, cucumber, collards, dandelion, beet leaves, chard, and celery
- Whole grains: brown, black, and wild rice; quinoa
- Hot peppers: cayenne, jalapeños, and habañeros
- Herbs and spices: turmeric, cinnamon, curry, ginger, licorice, ginseng, cilantro, rhodiola, basil, and ashwagandha

Foods from the Sea

- Plants: spirulina, chlorella, and kelp
- Cold-water fish: salmon, sardines, tuna, trout, and mackerel

SUPERHEALING RECOMMENDATION: FOODS TO EXCLUDE FROM YOUR DIET

Avoid the following foods, because they can wreak havoc in your body:

- **Trans fat.** Do you find it hard to believe that junk food that contains trans fat contributes to brain shrinkage as we age, whereas a diet rich in nutrients prevents the brain from aging? Researchers at three Oregon institutions conducted a brain-aging study, with participants whose average age was eighty-seven. The results showed that those with higher blood levels of vitamins E, D, C, and B and omega-3 fatty acids (primarily from fish) scored higher on memory and cognitive tests. Brain scans also showed they had larger brain volume at the end of the study, which means that they had less tissue shrinkage, than those who had more trans-fat in their bloodstreams.[26] This study was particularly credible, compared with projects that have relied on participants' subjective recollections recorded in food diaries, because the researchers measured the blood levels of the specific nutrients to get their results.

- **Genetically modified organisms (GMOs).** To date, GMOs have never been properly tested in humans or animals on a long-term basis, and since they are created through a violently disruptive process of gene splicing, they are suspect. When given the option, most animals avoid them. There are many questions about the effect of genetic modification on human health and the true need for these foods. For the time being, I do my best to avoid them. Most processed and fresh corn, if not labeled organic, is genetically modified.

- **Soy.** Many times during my childhood, I heard my relatives comment that soy wasn't good for humans. Now it turns out that one of the biggest myths in the health-food industry is that soy is good for you. This is a lie. The beans contain chemicals that suppress thyroid function.[27] And even though fermented soy products such as soy sauce, tempeh, and miso do contain lower levels of the health-damaging chemicals, I still advise against consuming them. Unfortunately, for a long time, I didn't know how detrimental soy could be, so I consumed large amounts of tofu, soy milk, soy burgers, soy ice cream, and soy cheeses. I have now amended my diet by cutting them out.

- **Artificial sweeteners and flavor enhancers.** As mentioned earlier, these cause brain damage, and flavorings are created to act like addictive substances to make you eat more of them. They cause such severe overstimulation of certain key areas of the brain that it can lead to their death. They have been implicated in the dramatic increase in a variety of neurological disorders, from attention deficit disorder in children to Parkinson's disease, Alzheimer's disease, multiple sclerosis, and brain tumors and dementia in adults.

SUPERHEALING RECOMMENDATION: NUTRITIONAL SUPPLEMENTS TO TAKE REGULARLY

It's a very good idea to take comprehensive vitamin and mineral supplements on a daily basis because of the significant decline in the last fifty years of the inherent nutrient value of the fruits and vegetables that are available to us.[28] The following supplements are particularly beneficial in activating our superhealing capabilities:

- **Omega-3 fatty acids.** These are known to reduce oxidative stress and inflammation, lengthen telomeres, and decrease the risk for major diseases associated with aging, such as heart disease, type 2 diabetes, arthritis, and Alzheimer's disease. Sources include fish oil capsules, flaxseed, chia seeds, walnuts, and pine nuts.[29]

- **Vitamin D$_3$.** A naturally occurring hormone in the body that is produced during exposure to sunlight, vitamin D$_3$ forms stronger bones, lowers blood pressure, prevents various cancers, improves muscle health, and increases metabolic activity in fat cells.[30]

- **Astaxanthin.** This has powerful antioxidant properties and is particularly beneficial to the joints, tendons, skin, eyes, and brain.[31] A carotenoid—which means it's in the same family as carrots and beets—it is derived from the microalgae *Haematococcus pluvialis.*

- **Resveratrol.** This nutrient compound is found in grape skins, blueberries, and red wine. It can improve motor coordination, protect nerve cells from deterioration caused by aging, cure type 2 diabetes, and fight inflammation and cancer.[32]

- **Theanine.** This is an amino acid found in green and black teas and in certain mushrooms. Preliminary research indicates that it is helpful in responding to stress, enhancing concentration, and possibly reducing the risk of stroke, Alzheimer's disease, and some forms of cancer.[33]

SUPERHEALING NUTRITION
ENGAGEMENT SUGGESTION

Write down everything you eat and maintain a food diary for seven to ten days. This will give you a much better understanding of your diet. There's a food diary in the Superhealing Workbook on my website.

SUPERHEALING WORK SHEET: ASSESSING YOUR DIET

Armed with the information contained in this chapter, consider these questions:

- Do you think you need to change your diet?
- How can you change your diet?
- Are you willing to eliminate or significantly reduce certain unhealthy foods?
- What healthy foods appeal to you?

Part Three

YOUR
SUPERHEALING
SPIRIT

CHAPTER 7

YOUR SUPERHEALING
SPIRIT-BODY CONNECTION

Be sure that it is not you that is mortal, but only your body.
For that man whom your outward form reveals is not yourself;
the spirit is the true self, not that physical figure
which can be pointed out by your finger.

—Cicero

THROUGHOUT THIS BOOK, MY CHALLENGE HAS BEEN TO WRITE about different aspects of being—mind, body, and spirit—in a way that provides an understanding of the distinction among them in some respects but that also makes clear they are not entirely separate. The unity of being is the truth.

The core ingredient in the superhealing formula, however, is the spirit. The Divine is the highest place within each of us, an all-powerful and all-encompassing energy that is first and foremost love, light, intelligence, and beauty. I believe that the spirit is an individualized expression of the Divine: the defining, primal force of life. And when we are aligned with the Divine, nothing is impossible for us.

This revelation was a moment that forever changed my life—and it occurred in my bathtub. In the process of studying the healing practice of the laying on of hands, I was learning how to transfer energy. That day's session had been particularly intense. As I stood over my teacher, transferring energy into her body, the energy roared through me so much so that at one point I felt light-headed and almost passed out.

At home that evening, I took a bath before going to bed. While relaxing in the hot water listening to soothing meditation music, I heard a sound that I can only describe as high-pitched energy. After it rang in my ears for a few seconds, I was not in my body anymore and was floating in an ocean of bliss.

I was still me, but more than I could ever have imagined. I felt like a drop in that ocean, but a drop that had no clear physical definition. I was in the midst of one of the most powerful moments of my life. I felt part of everything, large and small. Suddenly, for some unknown reason, fear entered my mind. Then I heard a loving voice. From my perspective, it spoke to me from above. A sweet, feminine voice, it said, "Don't worry; you are one with all things. Don't worry."

After that, I felt my consciousness rapidly descend back into my body as though it were being siphoned through a funnel. It was awesome!

For months, I tried to think my way back into that state. It consumed my thoughts. That eternal moment of divine ecstasy forever altered my sense of self and my understanding of life. I knew in a most powerful and meaningful way that there was more—much, much, more—to me and to life than I had previously understood.

I still recall that event with great wonder. Today it seems to have integrated quietly into my consciousness. I feel its joy, peace, and bliss as part of my ongoing awareness when I am in alignment with my spirit, when I am in harmony with my being, and when my thoughts, feelings, and emotions are reflective of the truth.

WHAT IS SPIRIT?

Spirit, in its infinite expression, is the divine doorway to who we truly are. The eternal essence of life that is at the core of our existence, it was alive before our birth and will live on after our death. It is created in the image and likeness of the Divine, it is the reflection of the Divine that is present in all of us, and it is our transcendent sense of connection to the Divine. We are divine sparks becoming and unfolding into greater expression.

My experience is that spirit extends my sense of self and enfolds all of life. It is not separate but inclusive and unifying. The higher states that spirit engenders are the foundation of that sense, because they are by their very nature aspects of the oneness of the Divine and all things.

Is there a difference between *spirit* and *soul*? I often use the terms interchangeably. In my humble opinion, they are both the Divine. I believe we are created, as everything else in the universe is, in the image and likeness of the all-knowing, all-loving, all-intelligent infinite. When we are aligned with the Divine, nothing is impossible for us. The Divine is the highest place within each of us, a powerful and encompassing energy that is love, light, intelligence, and beauty. It is all that is: everything.

We are spiritual beings having a human experience, not the other way around. Spirit gives our body intelligence, energy, and substance. It is the life-giving, driving force that gives birth to the magnificent body. What we know as birth and death are the transitions when spirit inhabits us and departs from us. If the spirit didn't engage with the body, we simply would not exist.

As the animating force, spirit fundamentally guides and directs our bodily functions primarily through the mind, brain, and heart, but all organ systems are involved. Spirit expresses itself in every aspect of our body's functioning. We're just not consciously aware of all of it.

As the primary aspect of being human, spirit is the guiding light that engages the mind and the body. Spirit is the blueprint of all physical life. We tend not to give much thought to how our spirits interact with our bodies. Yet our brains—in fact, our entire bodies—are first and foremost spiritual beings. Having a high state of spirit, aligning with it through the doorway of the mind, and consciously engaging with it gives our existence the greatest meaning and opportunity for living beyond the mundane, repetitive patterns that have entangled much of our awareness.

When spirit flows freely through our minds and into our bodies, we are aligned, and superhealing is expressing fully in us. That harmony of being is awe-inspiring.

The Qualities of Spirit

Spirit's aspects include joy, bliss, compassion, peace, intelligence, wisdom, intuition, selflessness, altruism, passion, beauty, appreciation, vitality, and love. When it comes to love, spirit expresses the highest of all states of being that reflect it. These states embrace kindness, forgiveness, courage, generosity, acceptance, understanding, patience, gratitude, optimism, integrity, and sincerity.

WHAT IS SPIRITUALITY?

Spirituality is our primary connection to, and relationship with, life itself. An inseparable aspect of our being, it is at the root of our quest for meaning in life. For this reason, the spiritual dimension is the ultimate determining factor in our lives. Spirituality is an innate sense of connection to something greater than ourselves that is sacred, divine, and wondrous.

Spirituality is centered in our awareness of spirit's inherent goodness and of our connection to the foundation and life-giving source of everything. It is living with an open, loving heart. I believe that this is the ultimate goal of all religious efforts in their quest to discover the Divine. Spirituality is often confined to our religious experience, but I believe that spirit is involved with every aspect of life on a moment-to-moment basis. It is intensely personal and unique to everyone.

There are many ways to engage your spirituality. There is no right or wrong way. Spirituality is what you determine it to be for you. Many discover spirituality through religious affiliation or through a relationship with the Divine independent of organized religion. Others find it through creative expression, the arts, music, nature, a quest for truth (spiritual or scientific), and practicing the principles and values considered significant and life-enhancing. Some have discovered a greater sense of spirituality in such mind-body practices as meditation, yoga, tai chi, and so forth. Our personal relationships can also be an expression of spirituality.

I'd like to share with you, for your consideration, my foundational exploration and personal thoughts on spirit, spirituality, and religion. Please understand that these thoughts are mine and mine alone. I am not seeking to convert you to my belief system; I simply want to share my views with the sincere hope that they will help you to uncover, review, understand, and clarify your own.

In my opinion, religion is a man-made construct of ideas, doctrines, practices, and beliefs that were designed to address the specific spiritual needs of an individual or a group of people at a particular point in time. It is established and incorporated into the existing culture in a way that supports the goals and objectives of that society. Religion is a vehicle through which spirituality can express itself in that culture.

I've often been asked why I talk about science and spirit as if there were no conflict between the two. Why do I use science to demonstrate the value of spirit and spirituality? The break occurred, as I mentioned earlier, during the turf war between church and science.

But it never happened in reality. Spirit has always guided our physiology through the vehicle of the mind. I see no separation, because the division that exists between spirituality and science is arbitrary and unnecessary.

Remarkable research has proven that immersing ourselves in positive emotions and attributes associated with the spirit—such as love, intelligence, beauty, joy, and compassion—dramatically enhances our health and well-being and gives life its greatest meaning. The positive emotions, values, attitudes, beliefs and, strengths that we acquire through spiritual practices contribute to our health and happiness. The engagement of spiritual practices improves the quality of life, increases the likelihood of survival, and contributes to illness being less severe.[1]

According to both spiritual traditions and scientific discoveries, we are all beings of energy. The body's atoms and molecules vibrate at certain frequencies and generate waves of energy. Uplifting states of awareness physiologically alter our bodies and minds and guide them into a higher level of functioning and health. These states also enhance our likelihood of recovering from serious illnesses, promote longevity, and generally improve our lives.

When we express spiritual qualities, our physiology changes. There is a biology of hope, a physiology of love, and a biochemistry of peace. That is how intimately the spirit interacts with the body. When we feel these states, they are not just in our spirits, they are actual physical states. When the autonomic nervous system experiences positive emotions such as enthusiasm, love, awe, and amusement, compared to being in a state of emotional neutrality, unique patterns of activation occur, indicating the existence of many physiologically distinct positive emotions.[2]

While I have already shared with you the concepts of positive psychology, I think we need to take a deeper look at it now, because expressing positive emotions is the doorway to aligning the mind and the spirit and thus the body, too. I see a continuum of emotions, from the highest to the lowest—from love to sadness—and positive emotions fall within that spectrum. All the spiritual qualities are reflective of positivity, but the research so far has focused more on what I would call the psychological, rather than the spiritual, aspects of human nature. Positive emotions are part of our spiritual expression. They are the key to actively experiencing superhealing on an ongoing basis.

Living in states of emotional well-being, happiness, joy, optimism, satisfaction, and other positive moods and having a sense of humor are all associated with a decreased death rate, among healthy people as well as those experiencing illness.[3]

Lower emotional states include anger, envy, fear, frustration, pessimism, impatience, doubt, guilt, despair, dishonesty, revenge, selfishness, ingratitude, intolerance, sorrow, shame, and prejudice. They have their place and should not be shunned, ignored, or suppressed; rather, they should be experienced and explored for the messages, potential growth, greater understanding, and awareness that all our emotions can bring. Some people have been misled to believe that being spiritual requires dwelling in positivity 100 percent of the time. Nothing could be further from the truth. Superhealing is living authentically and experiencing all the different emotions our experiences bring.

Spiritual well-being can reduce our chances of developing diseases through dampening the fight-or-flight response and the sympathetic nervous system and enhancing calmness and the parasympathetic nervous system. Spiritual well-being may decrease inflammation and blood clotting that is triggered by stress.[4] Well-being causes a reduction in death from heart disease. Similar to the relaxation response, it lowers the level of cortisol, a key stress hormone.

Accessing superhealing through heightened well-being can decrease your risk of developing disease by changing your response to stress through the autonomic nervous system and by enhancing parasympathetic stimulation, elevating heart rate variability, and lowering blood pressure. By maintaining a positive state of well-being, you may reduce your vulnerability to infectious diseases and also not generate as high a level of the stress-induced chemicals that are involved with inflammation and coagulation, which are associated with cardiovascular disease.

Many studies now indicate that optimists are healthier than pessimists. The most comprehensive review of research findings discovered that a sense of well-being and feeling positive rather than distressed or depressed does contribute to enhanced health and longevity. By following 5,000 college students for more than forty years, one study showed that the most pessimistic students lived shorter lives than the other students did. Another research project, which involved tracking 180 nuns throughout their adult lives, determined that those who wrote autobiographies in which they indicated that they had been positive in their twenties tended to live longer than those who had negative recollections of their earlier lives.[5] Several long-term studies have determined that pessimism, anxiety, depression, and a lack of enjoyment of one's daily activities are all linked to higher rates of disease and statistically significant shorter lives. This, the researchers concluded, is because of the effects of long-term negative thinking. Occasional negative thoughts that occur in the midst of ongoing positivity are not as harmful.

YOUR SUPERHEALING
SPIRIT-HEART-BRAIN CONNECTION

Have you ever felt your heart speaking to you? Have you ever considered its significance beyond pumping blood through your body? It is indeed a specialized muscle that is unique unto itself. "It is only with the heart that one can see rightly," said the author Antoine de Saint-Exupéry. "What is important is invisible to the eye."

From time immemorial and around the globe, the heart has been perceived as the seat of our emotions. Our ancestors believed that the heart is where they experienced the sensation of love and where intuition, gratitude, and wisdom abided. For some cultures, the heart was the location of consciousness and of the soul. The heart has always been associated with the highest—that is, spiritual—human qualities.

Until studies showed otherwise, however, scientists focused on the brain as the source of these experiences. Now there is research that has explored the activities through which the heart actively communicates with the brain, transferring emotion and influencing biochemical and electrical processing through the nervous system. These studies provided the foundation to explain how and why the heart affects our emotions, mental clarity, creativity, and empathetic states.

We also now know that through the powerful electromagnetic energy the heart generates with each beat, it actually communicates and informs the brain and other organs of our emotional states, because our heart rate varies in accordance with those states. The heart contains a highly complex nervous system that has the capacity to learn and maintain memories independently of the brain.

Surprising, too, is that the heart communicates with the brain in ways that significantly affect our perceptions and our reactions to the world. Studies have determined that the heart has its own unique

mechanisms that are frequently different from the directions received from the autonomic nervous system. The heart appeared to
send messages to the brain, which received the messages and followed their instructions.[6] More recently, neuroscientists discovered
nerve cells and pathways where messages from the heart to the brain
could stop or enhance the brain's electrical activity.[7]

PHYSIOLOGICAL COHERENCE

The pathway between spirit and body via positive emotions is
a recently discovered physiological state known as *coherence.* Our
hearts are affected by our feelings and emotions, which alter the
heart rate and form a heart rhythm pattern. This coherent pattern is
an indication of our body's quality of functioning. It allows the two
parts of our nervous system (sympathetic and parasympathetic) to
function effectively together in harmony. Perhaps this is the physiological basis of positive emotions.

Our negative emotions create a very different vibration and state
throughout the body. Emotional distress causes an erratic and unpredictable heart rate, which is considered *incoherent.* It is an indication that the two parts of our autonomic nervous system are functioning independently of each other rather than together. One part is
stimulating while the other is attempting to relax. This wastes energy
and causes additional physical deterioration. This is especially true if
we experience stress and negative emotions on a regular basis.

SPIRITUALITY, HEALTH, AND WELL-BEING

As we consider the link between spirituality and health, I want to
be clear at the outset about something. *By no means is this intended
to make you feel less spiritual if you are living with an illness.*

Spirituality and health is the final medical frontier, yet to be fully explored and understood. And I believe it is one of the most important frontiers. When I was in medical school, there was never, and I do mean *never*, a conversation about the topic. However, it has proved to be one of the most promising areas of medical research for those daring enough to investigate. Fortunately, there are more and more research scientists who are boldly going where few others have previously dared to go.

A global survey of more than 132 countries and 136,000 people found that even though increased income (both personal and national) enhances life satisfaction, it does not automatically lead to a greater sense of personal well-being. The data revealed that positive feelings are more closely associated with having social support, fulfilling work, autonomy, and respect. This is the first global study to examine life satisfaction, daily emotional states, and the perspective that one's life is going well.[8]

Contrary to popular opinion, our well-being is not improved by the external signs of success that many cultures honor. Fame and wealth do not help with pain. However, enhancing our spirituality and spiritual well-being does, and it leads to greater self-awareness and happiness.

The basis of our spiritual health and well-being is becoming one with life itself through the awareness of our inseparable connection to everyone and everything. It is escaping the unconsciously self-imposed constraints of our ego identity: the constricted individualized personality we have become through the portal of our culture's ideas of who we should be rather than the truth of who we are.

There are three generally accepted areas of spiritual health and development:

1. The realization of our potential
2. The meaning and purpose of life
3. Internal happiness

The Realization of Our Potential

It is well documented that during our lifetimes, we experience stages of human awareness—a pathway of spiritual unfolding and well-being. First there is the narrowly bound focus on the self-interest of the ego, which is reactive to the external world and seeks to control it. Along the path, those boundaries soften as we develop a consideration of the needs of others. Ultimately, the boundaries expand to include our souls and all of life itself. This is truly the transformation of ego and personality to the spiritual reality of who we are. This pathway is the superhealing journey to optimal health and well-being, the most direct route to having all that you desire.

The Meaning and Purpose of Life

Taking a deeper look into our spirits and spirituality promotes a state of well-being in which we have a broader view of life that supports the expression of our full potential, the understanding of our purpose and the meaning of life, and the internal focus that promotes happiness from within.

Internal Happiness

As we grow into greater self awareness, we begin to experience positive spiritual qualities more often, from occasionally to regularly to continuously. We become more purposeful, resourceful, compassionate, giving, intuitive, spiritual, joyful, happy, and peaceful, and we experience negative emotions less frequently.

FAITH AND FORTITUDE

You've probably heard the saying that the difference between a pessimist and an optimist is that the pessimist sees a glass as half empty and the optimist sees the glass as half full. Just as pessimism leads to complacency and indecision, optimism leads to hope and self-actualization. According to *Merriam-Webster's Collegiate Dictionary*, optimism is "an inclination to put the most favorable construction upon actions and events or to anticipate the best possible outcome."

Faith brings a new dimension to the optimist-pessimist story. The difference between faith and optimism is that when the glass is completely empty, the optimist is likely to become a pessimist, but those who have faith remain optimistic.

Faith brings to optimism the belief in an unwavering potential. In the face of hopelessness, as in the case of the empty glass, faith transcends the limits of logic and ego. Faith emerges from within your spirit and is reflective of a deeper belief and trust in the Divine. Optimism, however, is more a function of your personality. Traditionally, faith is considered to be the substance of things hoped for, the evidence of things not seen. It is our link to the greater mind, to the infinite field of possibilities, to the Divine. Faith in tomorrow, faith in the often unseen goodness that surrounds us, and faith in the Divine and in ourselves make life bearable in challenging times.

My experiences with people in the midst of confronting and curing a vast array of diseases made me aware of many universal traits and characteristics in those who experienced healing. They commonly share three qualities during the process: faith, fortitude, and forgiveness. We'll explore faith and fortitude here and take a look into forgiveness in the next chapter.

Faith

The first questions I ask when someone approaches me for help with a life-threatening condition such as cancer are "Do you want to live?" and "Why?" I also ask the relatives whether their loved one has lost the will to live.

Because faith engenders hope, it is the fuel that gives life to the will. It transcends belief and is reflective of an intuitive knowing of the truth that persists in the face of contradictory evidence. Faith transcends the realities of our existence. It cultivates hope and a spirit of renewal. It is a direct link to the field of infinite possibilities that dwells in the spirit.

The capacity to express faith in various degrees is probably the most common quality I have seen in patients who overcome and heal from life-threatening illnesses. I believe that faith stimulates physiological changes that promote superhealing. Yet faith must be distinguished from false hope. Faith emerges from the spirit, whereas false hope resides in the ego.

Because faith is born of the spirit, it is accepting and does not deny reality. It merely sees beyond it. Faith is a manifestation of the will to live. Many times during the years of my medical practice, I've had the privilege of treating patients who possessed unbelievable amounts of faith in the midst of seemingly hopeless situations.

Fortitude

The ability to persevere in the face of significant adversity is fortitude's key element. Fortitude is faith in action, and it arises from the spirit. Positive emotions fertilize and support the development of fortitude.

I am always amazed by the resilience and fortitude of children. It seems the younger they are, the greater access they have to superhealing. One of the most moving experiences I've ever had, with the patient who has affected me the most, occurred during my final days of medical school. Yolanda was a baby girl who has vibrantly remained at the forefront of my memory.

Yolanda's mother suddenly went into labor during the seventh month of pregnancy. At that time, the mid-1970s, there was no medication to reverse the process. Before Yolanda was born, the obstetrician knew that the chances of her survival were nonexistent.

Yolanda was extremely premature, weighing less than two and a half pounds. When she was born, she exhibited only a few signs of life, indicating that she was in severe physical distress. Her heartbeat was barely noticeable, and her breathing consisted of shallow, erratic grunts. Considering her size and the fact that no baby as premature as she had ever survived, the attending obstetrician informed her parents that their baby girl had been born dead.

After the delivery, the staff followed routine procedures, notifying the pathology department that the baby's body had to be picked up for an autopsy. For hours, she remained all alone in that cold, dark room. But unbeknownst to anyone, little Yolanda was clinging to life, one gasp of air at a time.

When the technician arrived much later to collect her body, he was shocked to discover a breathing baby! He notified the doctors on call that evening in the hospital's intensive-care nursery. In light of her severe prematurity and extreme condition, the doctors made a decision not to vigorously resuscitate her or provide her with the care she desperately needed. The doctors were certain that she wouldn't make it through that night, since several critical hours had lapsed between her birth and her arrival at the unit. During the night, she was given only minimal life support, oxygen through a hood instead of a respirator, and an IV instead of an arterial line that could have more easily monitored her condition.

The next morning, Yolanda was still alive and kicking, much to the shock of the staff in the nursery. Since her vital signs had slightly improved and she had remained pretty stable throughout the night, a decision was made concerning her care, as well as what to tell her parents, since they were still grieving her death.

The obstetrician who had delivered her and the pediatrician in charge of the nursery visited her mother's room that morning. Together they told the parents that their little girl was alive by virtue of an act of God. The doctors also informed them that she would receive the intensive medical care that she needed. But they also gave the parents very little realistic hope of her survival, warning them that she'd probably live no longer than a few more hours or days, at most. The doctors told the parents not to expect to ever take their baby home from the hospital.

Despite the physicians' appropriate reservations, no holds were barred from that moment forward. Yolanda was placed on complete life support: a respirator, a heart monitor, an umbilical artery catheter, and the appropriate medication.

Throughout the first few weeks of her life, Yolanda was never more than a breath away from death. Her vital signs were tenuous at best. One severe complication and crisis ensued after another, arising with unbelievable regularity. Despite such extreme challenges, Yolanda simply refused to die. Over the weeks and months that followed, she very slowly began to improve, valiantly fighting off and surviving a succession of life-threatening conditions, from bleeding in her brain to intestinal obstruction requiring surgery, from a heart defect that wouldn't resolve on its own to infection. She conquered several brain hemorrhages and brain-damaging jaundice, required repeated blood transfusions, and incurred lung damage from her prolonged exposure to high oxygen levels while she was on the ventilator. Yolanda's spirit never allowed death's ever-present shadow to conquer her tiny body and indomitable will to live.

Her improvements slowly grew beyond the minute incremental

ones that initially occurred. She began to gain more weight, strengthening her reserves. She began to respond to her environment, smiling at her parents and nurses, suckling and cooing, but at a much slower pace compared to normal babies. Gradually she started to grasp her nurse's fingers.

There was a moment of celebration in the nursery the day Yolanda held a small toy in her hand. The infections ceased, the internal bleeding in her brain stopped, and the transfusions were no longer necessary. And with great difficulty she was tenaciously weaned from the respirator that had acted as her lungs for so many months.

I was privileged to be on call the Sunday afternoon Yolanda was discharged from the hospital. After a six-month battle, she had defied and defeated the significant odds against her, as well as her doctors' realistically grim predictions, and she went home with her parents. It was the highlight of my years in medical school, a thrilling moment that will remain vividly implanted in my memory for the rest of my life. It was touching, emotional, and uniquely rewarding to see that little girl face and overcome a seemingly infinite number of insurmountable obstacles in six months.

Yolanda has given me courage, faith, strength, and a profound appreciation of how indomitable the human spirit truly is. It can survive anything. In ny own moments of weakness, the memory of Yolanda has come to me spontaneously. Sometimes I wonder where she is and how life is treating her. Yolanda is just one of the patients who clearly demonstrated to me the powerful role that fortitude—the will to live—plays in engaging superhealing.

Fortitude allows us to face life with confidence. It is a resilient determination that springs forth from our spirits, not from circumstances. It prevents us from succumbing to the tragic episodes of life and is the substance of the will to live.

CHAPTER 8

THE SUPERHEALING POWER
OF LOVE AND RELATIONSHIPS

Love is the most powerful force in the world,
yet it is the humblest imaginable.

—Mahatma Gandhi

ALL THE TECHNIQUES AND INFORMATION I'VE SHARED WITH YOU
throughout the course of this book rest on the foundational reality that superhealing comes from the Divine, which is expressed through our essence, the spirit. And love is the primary source of the spirit, the creative substance from which all other aspects of the spirit flow. It is the most important force in the universe. There are no limitations to love, and after all other things have ended, love will remain, never ceasing. In short, love makes the world go around.

Love is the light that gives us life, and we are created in its image. At the core of our being, where peace, joy, bliss, mercy, grace, and compassion abide, we are all essentially good, loving, and lovable. That is true regardless of what we tell ourselves or what the rest of the world might tell us. Love is the source of meaning and inspiration. It is the intelligence that allows us to rise above our existing patterns of thought and behavior to connect, to forgive, to be grateful, to be charitable, and to make choices beyond experiences that cause stress. Love is the key ingredient to living life well. Without our awareness and expression of it, our lives are but a shadow of what they could be.

We all need love, regardless of who we are and our position or status. The external substitutes for love—material possessions, money, power, position, prestige, and so forth—are poor replacements for the rich gifts of the spirit. These things have their place, and you do not need to abandon them, but perhaps you should reconsider the context in which you view them.

You might be wondering what love has to do with superhealing. The answer is everything! At its core, superhealing is an expression of love. It's been said that there are only two true emotions, love and fear, with variations therein. When we are not in a state of love, we're dwelling in fear. Fear is what causes our distress and increases our likelihood of becoming ill. Love can elevate our consciousness from where it currently resides to a place of healing and reformation. It's the source of the miracles, magic, and wonder that give meaning to life and liberate us from disease, despair, isolation, and rejection. Modern medicine is, perhaps, finally beginning to recognize the role that love plays in our well-being. Babies die without it, children's growth and development require it, and adults need it to enhance their purpose and meaning in life.

In this chapter, I address self-love, which is activated by attention, awareness, and acceptance; the healing power of loving touch; how relationships are a central component of superhealing; and the health benefits of altruism, gratitude, and forgiveness. All these various expressions of love are important keys to superhealing.

SELF-LOVE AND COMPASSION

I believe that the most significant and important relationship we have in our life is often overlooked. It's the one we have with ourselves and the Divine that resides within us. Ultimately, superhealing is loving ourselves with total self-acceptance: being fine with who we are just the way we are. When we get that right, we are right with the world.

Self-love is flexible, kind, giving, compassionate, and understanding. It is the basis for all the love we give to and share with others. When we love ourselves, our minds, bodies, and spirits are in harmony and express a high-functioning physiology, both physically and emotionally.

Yet many of us were born into families that did not know how to help us develop our awareness of all the love that dwells inside us. As children, we are often encouraged to become externally focused and to disregard our internal messages, dialogue, and guidance. That leads to the fear and self-doubt that ultimately results in self-disregard. I also believe it is difficult to love ourselves in the vacuum created by not relating love to our spirituality.

How do we set that right? I've heard patients ask, "How do I begin to love myself? What do you mean? I feel so unworthy! I've known how to love others, but not myself. Where do I start?"

True self-love is always present; we only need to remove the disharmony that is preventing its expression. Nothing has to be different for us to be whole. It is a matter of changing our perspectives and perceptions.

One of the easiest ways to begin is to start to pay attention to yourself. Attention is the act of applying the mind to something with awareness—you, in this case. Listen to your inner voice and to what you are saying to yourself. We often speak more negatively to ourselves than we ever would to anyone else. Usually, we criticize ourselves more than we praise ourselves.

Some in our culture would argue that to focus on and nurture ourselves is to be selfish. Self-love is often confused with narcissism. Narcissism, or self-centeredness, is the opposite of self-love. It is demanding, immature, and unrelenting. Narcissists are compensating for a falsely perceived sense of their own inferiority. Arrogance and selfishness are outward manifestations of fear and insecurity. Narcissism seeks to soothe our pain, but it is a poor and incapable substitute for self-love. It tries to gain from the outer world something that only the inner world can provide. A secure soul, in contrast to a narcissistic one, is open and loving.

Learning to love yourself, however, doesn't mean that from then on everything will always come up roses. Difficulties will persist, and sometimes they become even greater. The sign of our growth is not the absence of difficulties but the way we handle them. The superhealing that comes from loving ourselves softens our negativity, loosening its grasp. We take responsibility. We make conscious and unconscious choices of how to respond to any situation.

Self-love is the portal to superhealing, which comes not from us but through us. That portal leads to a pathway with no ultimate destination, since there is no endpoint to your optimal health and wellbeing. Like a blossoming flower, it continuously unfolds from the center of your being and occurs in its own way and own time.

Superhealing is unique to each of us. For a few, the alignment that leads to superhealing occurs quickly, even spontaneously. More commonly, though, it takes months, years, and sometimes decades. And even when it does occur suddenly, it's truly just the beginning, an initiating event of sorts.

What about the past? How does everything that we have done before now affect the present? The past is over. Let it go. There is no need for guilt or blame, only for understanding and healing. One day, perhaps even sooner than you can imagine now, you will become more appreciative of the lessons that past events afforded you, as difficult and challenging as they might have been at the time.

The path of superhealing guides us to our primary and inseparable wholeness, the core of our being. Peace of mind, self-acceptance, and knowledge of one's true nature comes from living in tune with one's inner self and experiencing the spirit within. To be whole is to be complete, to be all-encompassing.

THE SUPERHEALING POWER OF TOUCH

Skin is our body's largest organ, containing millions of nerve receptor cells, and touch is the first sensation we experience, beginning in the womb long before we are born. Touch is a primal form of communication, a formidable and fundamental ingredient of our humanity. Indeed, perhaps it's the most critical element of our humanity, integral to every intimate, emotionally involved relationship we have. The vehicle for sharing love, kindness, and support, touch is a vital to human expression and interaction.

Touch is not limited to our relationships with other people but extends to those with animals as well. Something amazing occurred with rabbits in a study at Ohio State University that baffled the researchers. The rabbits were being fed a high-fat diet to test a new cholesterol-lowering drug. Based on earlier findings, the researchers expected highly predictable results. But this was not the case. Despite their unhealthy diet, certain rabbits had no sign of heart disease. The scientists couldn't figure out why; they didn't have a clue what was going on in their own lab.

The researchers had anticipated that there would be some lessening of atherosclerosis (hardening of the arteries) because of the drug, but they had never seen animals fed such a high-fat diet show not even minimal signs of heart disease. By comparing the disease-free rabbits to the other rabbits that were on the same regimen, they knew it wasn't genetic. Nor was it was due to their sex; some were male and some were female.

So what caused these particular rabbits to not develop heart disease in a tightly controlled and monitored lab setting? What factor defied the expectations? The researchers conducted a painstaking review of the procedures and of everything that had happened to these rabbits. They couldn't or wouldn't believe the apparent reason. Here's what stymied them.

The rabbits were kept in rows of cages stacked on top of one another. The lab technician who fed them was a short woman, and the researchers discovered that she would take only the rabbits on the lower tier out of their cages and hold them, pet them, and talk to them while they ate. No one wanted to believe that loving the rabbits while they ate would affect their physiology as dramatically as it did. So the researchers repeated the test twice more and got the same results. The petting continued to be the sole protective factor.[1]

Something profound happened to the petted animals. I believe it is compelling evidence of the power of love. The feeling of being loved that they got from the lab technician's demonstrations of attention and affection changed their physiology despite the fact that they were not living a normal rabbit's life. Those few moments of petting while eating a very damaging diet altered their physiology in a very positive way.

Years earlier, I was intrigued by a similarly fascinating study about touch. During my junior year in college, while taking a child psychology course, I learned something that to this day continues to haunt me with awe and sadness. Baby primates and humans will die if they are not touched, even if they receive proper nutrition. They wither away from a condition known as *failure to thrive*.

Being touched lovingly can reduce one's blood pressure, heart rate, and cortisol level and can trigger the release of oxytocin, the bonding hormone, and endorphins, the natural opiates that help the body's cells function more efficiently.[2]

The Touch Research Institute at the University of Miami School of Medicine has conducted more than 100 studies on touch and discovered proof of its significant health-enhancing effects, including weight gain and growth in premature babies, improved functioning of cancer patients' immune systems, reduced pain, lower glucose (sugar) levels in diabetic children, and decreased autoimmune disease symptoms.[3]

Other studies have scientifically determined that emotions can be expressed by touch. Researchers at DePaul University in Indiana evaluated people being touched by strangers they could not see. The one doing the touching was directed to attempt to communicate a particular emotion, and the majority of those being touched were able to accurately determine the emotional state of the toucher. This suggests that we can communicate several distinct emotions through touch: love, gratitude, anger, disgust, fear, and sympathy.[4] This study also suggests that touch is a much more meaningful method of communication than previously considered. It may be that touch heals but that it needs the person doing the touching to be in the right mood. That may explain why a mother's hug can literally "make it better." How often do mothers say, "Let me kiss it and make it better" when their children skin their knees?

The United States has been found to be one of the cultures with the least amount of touching, compared to others. For example, Dr. Tiffany Field and associates at the Touch Research Institute observed teenagers at McDonald's restaurants in Miami and Paris to measure how much they touched and engaged in aggressive behavior during their interactions. American teens spent much less time touching, embracing, and stroking their friends compared to their French counterparts, although they engaged in more self-touching. The Americans were also more physically and verbally aggressive.[5] Preschool children in the two countries were then observed while playing outside with their friends and their parents. Again, the American children were more aggressive toward both their parents and their friends and touched them less.[6]

THE POWER OF LOVING RELATIONSHIPS

While touch is a powerful aspect of our communication with others, our relationships are also central to superhealing. We exist in a relational universe—that is, everything exists in relation to everything else—and this framework gives meaning and perspective to life.

As a species, humans are social beings. (This also applies to some animals, such as elephants and dolphins.) Relationships are the fundamental way we express love, and it has been proved that healthy relationships have a tremendous positive effect on our well-being. Isolation and adversarial relationships contribute to physical decline and psychological turmoil.

From the moment of conception to the time of death, relationships are a pervasive and encompassing part of life, serving many important functions. Social isolation is a significant health risk. Researchers made a dramatic finding in the 1980s when, after following thousands of residents of Alameda County, California, for several years, they determined social isolation to be a significant risk factor for all diseases, including heart disease. Since then, other scientists around the world have confirmed a link between lack of social support and the development of heart disease in humans and animals.[7]

Did you know that supportive relationships are the strongest predictor of good health thoughout the course of our lives? Family ties and friendships enhance our health and exert one of the most potent protective mechanisms against the development of disease. Examples abound, from the healing power of social support to the benefits of a happy marriage.

A study of patients recovering from heart attacks found that those with lower amounts of emotional support were nearly three times as likely to die in six months as those with higher levels of emotional support.[8] Social support is linked to lower death rates from a variety of other diseases, and there is relatively strong evidence linking it to aspects of the functioning of the cardiovascular, endocrine, and immune systems. Death from conditions of these systems occurs more often among people who are isolated. In fact, isolation is considered to be a comparable risk factor to smoking, a sedentary lifestyle, and high blood pressure. The quantity and quality of our social relationships are related not only to the prevention of disease but also to longevity. Isolation was defined as being physically apart, i.e., separated from others to the extreme. While there are certainly people who prefer to be alone, most don't, and the physical and perception of separation from others and the absence of emotional support, are powerful determinants of health.

Studies have shown that in general, married people tend to be healthier and happier than those who are single.[9] For example, a supportive, happy marriage is linked with greater longevity after a diagnosis of a life-threatening illness, faster recovery from an injury, and a lower risk of infection.[10] A loving wife is also associated with a decreased risk of men developing ulcers.[11] In another study, a wife's love was associated with a 50 percent reduction of angina (chest pain) compared with that experienced by those who felt unloved and unsupported.[12]

Depression is a significant risk factor for coronary artery disease and heart attacks. Studies have looked at participation in voluntary associations and religious groups, the number of close friendships, and the distance from one's primary source of support as significant predictors of the development of the symptoms of depression.

Depression has been linked to the size of a person's social network; the fewer the number of friends, the greater the chance of developing depression.[13] Studies on the health-enhancing value of support groups have documented their positive effects on reversing heart disease (in conjunction with diet modification, relaxation, and physical activity) and on extending life in terminally ill cancer patients.[14]

One of the most fascinating studies I've ever read involved the residents of Roseto, a small town in Pennsylvania. Early in the 1960s, this small town became well-known to the national medical community because the residents had a very low incidence of heart disease despite the fact that they ate a high-fat, high-cholesterol diet and drank alcohol on a regular basis. Researchers sought to discover the cause of this unusual phenomenon and concluded that the supportive, interactive, and close-knit nature of the town's primarily Italian American population created an immunity to heart disease. The protection from heart disease occurred because these immigrants still maintained an Italian lifestyle, including very strong familial and social ties.

Researchers predicted that the rate of heart disease would increase as the town's citizens adopted a more Americanized lifestyle, and that is exactly what they found when they returned in the mid-1970s. During the 1980s, cholesterol education programs and other public health measures lowered the incidence of heart disease nationally. However, when researchers returned to Roseto yet again in 1985, they found that despite decreases in fat intake and the smoking rate among its inhabitants, the occurrence of heart disease continued to climb there. They concluded that the population's assimilation of American-style conspicuous consumption and materialism had prevented the expected decline in heart disease.[15]

Japanese culture is also characterized by a high degree of social support. There is evidence that this may contribute to the low rate of heart disease in Japan and among Japanese Americans, who, as their Italian American counterparts in Roseto once did, still retain their traditional culture.

All this research suggesting that the coming together and breaking apart of social relationships have important physiological consequences in humans and other animals. Creating and sustaining supportive and enduring relationships triggers reward pathways in our brains that allow love to motivate and delight us. They also suppress the pathways that make us more judgmental and likely to experience negative emotions.

It hurts most when we are rejected—both when we reject ourselves and when others do it to us. In fact, social pain is relieved by the same drugs that relieve physical pain, because the pathways that cause physical and emotional pain overlap in our brains.[16]

So it should come as no surprise that healthy relationships are a cornerstone of our well-being; they improve our lives significantly, not only emotionally but physically as well. Social bonding and soothing behaviors relieve the damaging effects of negative events and enhance our health. Healthy relationships buffer us from the stresses of life and diminish the stress response and activity in the autonomic nervous system and the hypothalamic-pituitary-adrenal axis—the endocrine system that responds to stress, by releasing hormones that instruct our cells to change their normal functioning and prepare to run or fight.[17] Our sense of connection to others helps to diminish our usual response to stress and to pain.[18]

ALTRUISM AND SELFLESS GIVING

My parents were deeply spiritual and religious people. Growing up with parents whose lives were integrated with their spiritual beliefs, which included helping others, I didn't analyze the health benefits of volunteerism. But I did watch them live it and was often moved by their integrity, kindness, and consideration of others. They were very family oriented, and "family" extended beyond the nuclear unit. They taught me to see our family as part of the larger family of humanity. They never met a stranger, as they welcomed and treated newcomers as if they'd known them for many years, and they opened the doors of our home to everyone.

My parents frequently performed quiet random acts of kindness: giving to children in our neighborhood and helping out neighbors and friends. My mother often cooked meals for homebound senior citizens, and my father gave his homegrown organic vegetables to many people. My parents were my great examples of how to be kind and live a good, loving life. They set the example for my own spiritual path and growth.

I still vividly remember an incident while I was grocery shopping with my father when I was seven years old. My father noticed a visibly distressed elderly woman who was crying and talking to the manager of the store. Though listening patiently, the manager did not appear to be moved by this woman's tears. I watched as my father approached them, exchanged a few words, opened his wallet, and handed the woman several dollars. I saw relief wash over her face. She grasped Daddy's hand and profusely thanked him. He smiled gently and said, "You're welcome, ma'am" as he walked away.

We went about our business. Daddy didn't say a word, but I wanted to know what had happened. On the way home, I asked, "Daddy what was wrong with that lady?"

"She got off the bus and left her purse on it," he explained. "She didn't have a way to get home, so I gave her a few dollars to make sure that she did and to get something to eat." Back then a bus ride cost fifteen or twenty cents.

As a young child, I was taken with not only his generosity but also his humility. It was no big deal to him, and he didn't brag. He was very matter-of-fact about it. That was the first random act of kindness I clearly recall witnessing. I never forgot what Daddy did that day, or his humility. That one experience affected me deeply, and I've used it as a model and a guide for including altruism in my life.

Altruism is internally motivated behavior that is born from a concern for the welfare of others rather than the anticipation of a benefit or reward. Our health and well-being benefit from helping others, if we can give without stressing and wearing ourselves out. There can be consequences to giving too much. Giving is beneficial only up to the point that it becomes physically and psychologically taxing. In other words, take care of yourself while you're taking care of others.

Many volunteers report that they experience well-being, increased energy, warmth, and pain reduction as well as increased optimism and self-esteem. The afterglow that comes from performing altruistic acts, sometimes called "helper's high," can last from one hour to the rest of the entire day. There was a survey of 3,000 volunteers who regularly put in two hours per week, an average of eight hours a month, helping others. All of them had personal contact with the strangers they helped, and 71 percent of them reported feelings of well-being similar to the high described by long-distance runners.[19]

Volunteering and support groups both appear to stimulate changes in our bodily functions similar to those researchers have observed occurring during meditation—that is, the relaxation response. Volunteering could well be considered a relaxation technique, since it disrupts self-focused thoughts and decreases the adrenal stress that occurs with the fight-or-flight response. Volunteering is beneficial in a variety of other ways, too: It improves our mood, distracts us from our problems and puts them into a broader perspective, creates enhanced meaning in life, increases our perception of our own effectiveness, and improves our social interactions. This all bears out the old adage that it's better to give than to receive—especially when it's done selflessly.

I wasn't surprised to discover that volunteering has all these health benefits. But the key to achieving them is to not seek the benefits but to give from your heart. There's a broad spectrum of reasons for volunteering, from those that are selfless to those that are self-serving. In one study, people who volunteered out of a desire to help others were found to live longer compared to those who volunteered for self-oriented reasons and to nonvolunteers.[20] Another study compared a group of senior citizen volunteers who gave massages to infants with a control group engaged in self-massage, and it found that the volunteers experienced lower levels of stress hormones and less anxiety than the others.[21]

Perhaps these findings are reflective of the spiritual belief that becoming lovingly other-focused is the highest state of being.

GRATITUDE

One of the most powerful superhealing techniques in existence is the expression of gratitude. Researchers give multiple definitions of *gratitude* in their studies. The word comes from the Latin *gratus*, meaning "agreeable" and "pleasing." I use *gratitude* and *appreciation* interchangeably. But gratitude, by any definition, enhances our sense of well-being, lifting us up to a state of superhealing in which our spirit, mind, and body are aligned and functioning in a harmonious state. When our hearts are open and giving thanks, it's as though the floodgates have opened.

Being grateful emphasizes the positive and releases the hold that negative thought tends to have on the mind. Gratitude uplifts the spirit and is an expression of love. It improves physical and psychological health and increases participation in healthy activities. It makes life sweeter and easier.

By increasing our vitality, gratitude helps us to feel alive and engaged. Our bodies transform in response. Like other positive emotions, gratitude helps the heart to function more efficiently by creating harmony between the heartbeat and the nervous system. Subsequently, all other bodily functions harmonize with this, and we experience coherence. As noted earlier, coherence leads to improved brain functioning, mental clarity, and creativity, among other enhanced functions.

Expressing gratitude makes us happier and more resistant to the unpleasant emotions that fuel stress, such as envy, anger, resentment, and regret. If we do experience stress, gratitude blunts and buffers the impact of it. When we are grateful, we have greater peace of mind and are even better at problem solving and decision making.[22]

According to one study, expressing gratitude to others is good for both you and the person being thanked. It can powerfully uplift a relationship mired in negativity, shifting our focus from what is wrong to what is right in the relationship and leading to a more positive and healthier connection. We can sometimes become unconscious of the full power and meaning of our relationships. In our busy, hectic lives, we often forget and overlook the significance of the people whose presence adds meaning to our lives. Expressing gratitude to them plays a pivotal role in the development and sustaining of our relationships and supports behaviors that are inclusive.[23;]

FORGIVENESS

Forgiveness is a foundational aspect of all religions and spiritual practices. Although ancient scriptures implore us to forgive others, it is one of the hardest yet most rewarding of all human challenges.

Forgiveness is truly one of the most taxing aspects of superhealing, but in order to achieve superhealing, we must forgive. Superhealing and anger cannot occupy the same space. Type A personalities are usually characterized as competitive and driven and as having a higher risk of heart attacks. But researchers say that this risk is a result of their hostility and unresolved anger rather than their personality traits.

We tend to believe that forgiveness supports the transgression that has been committed against us. But forgiveness is not an endorsement of wrongdoing; rather, it's an act of releasing the pain and hurt it caused through love, the root of forgiveness—and it is not love of the other but of the self. We must forgive ourselves as well as others in order to be whole and healed. Let me explain.

Forgiveness provides physiological relief from entangled and painful memories, releasing the ties that have bound us to the past and allowing us to move on. These old, unresolved wounds are the energetic, emotional dams that prevent the unobstructed flow of superhealing into our lives. We must forgive ourselves for our own transgressions. Forgiveness aids in the process of healing self-abuse and self-hatred. We must bring unhealed wounds out of the shadows. We cannot truly love ourselves without forgiveness. Once we begin to forgive ourselves, we can forgive others.

We can often be more forgiving of others than of ourselves. Still, how do we begin to forgive those who have caused us great pain? It isn't easy, but it is imperative. When we open our hearts to the idea of forgiveness, the areas that we need to forgive the most are not usually the wrongdoings that first come to mind, but the deeper hidden transgressions. Because they are so severe, they tend to surface gradually.

Many of us have made our way through life avoiding and suppressing our pain rather than confronting it. Breakthroughs occur after months or years of therapy, when painful memories come to the surface. When those wounds are healed, forgiving transformations occur. We often feel less slighted, less inadequate, and more loving.

John (not his real name), a young man in his early twenties, was prompted to see me because of a severe case of ulcers. His pain was minimally improved by medication, and he refused to have surgery. We approached his treatment from a superhealing perspective, and over the course of several months, some of his symptoms lessened, but there was no significant resolution of his condition.

He was extremely resistant to resolving his emotional issues and wanted to focus entirely on healing his physical symptoms—that is, until one session during meditation, when memories of severe abuse by his father in his early childhood flooded his mind. He had not been consciously aware of these incidents, although he knew he held a deep resentment and anger toward his father.

In the months that followed, John began to consciously confront and heal the old wounds and pain in concert with facing his father and attempting to repair their relationship. His father initially denied ever abusing him, but then he finally admitted it. John's ulcer began to rapidly improve during this period of emotional healing. His symptoms disappeared, and he was able to discontinue his medication and treatment.

✳✳✳

In lieu of a work sheet for this section, please review your answers about your relationships on the Life Inventory work sheet in the Introduction.

CHAPTER 9

ENGAGING YOUR SUPERHEALING SPIRIT

Before enlightenment, chop wood, carry water.
After enlightenment, chop wood, carry water.

—*Zen proverb*

SOME YEARS AGO WHILE WALKING THROUGH THE PARKING LOT OF A major big box store, I saw a beautiful little boy sitting in a shopping cart being pushed by his mother. His arms were outstretched as if to embrace everyone in his presence, and as they approached me, he turned his joyful smile in my direction. As he looked at me, beaming, he held out his arms toward me. I felt his heart embracing me, as though he'd actually wrapped his arms around me, and I also felt my heart returning his embrace.

It all happened in just a few seconds, but it was a powerful and beautiful moment that I will never forget.

His mother looked and me and said, "He's like this everywhere we go. He just wants to love the world. It's so embarrassing."

"Don't be embarrassed," I replied. "He's beautiful."

I believe babies and young children are our purest and most accessible example of spiritual engagement. They live entirely in the moment and are always express their truth. Upset one moment, they can become happy with lightning speed. It's not until much later in life that we linger in sadness.

Children haven't experienced enough involvement with the external world to displace their natural awareness of love, and they are naturally and openly connected to their spirits. There are no prolonged interfering thoughts or emotions that separate them from their spirits. They remind us of who we are and of the beauty that lies within us. Over time, however, that engagement with spirit dwindles, and as adults, we shift our focus to the physical realm. Still, spirit remains the core of our being and waits for our conscious return to it.

Since the dawn of civilization and throughout antiquity, teachers and priests encouraged an initiate to "know thyself." To know ourselves means knowing that our spirit is our essence that expresses itself through the mind and manifests as the body. Actively engaging ourspirit is the most direct pathway to discovering our essence and unfolding who we really are.

Our spirits long for greater expression, recognition, and conscious engagement in our daily lives. This calls for reconsidering our sense of purpose and enhances the meaning and rewards of life. Engaging our spirit fosters a growing awareness, an honesty of perception, and an acceptance of what is. The more we nurture our spirit, the more we will experience greater harmony and joy of being.

Engaging with our spirit allows us the opportunity to obtain a greater knowledge of our inner being and a broader appreciation for and understanding of our lives and our world. It is the primary doorway to health and well-being if we want to resolve an illness or an imbalance. I also believe that it will lead us to the manifestation of the world we desire. Mahatma Gandhi is quoted as saying, "If we could change ourselves, the tendencies in the world would also change."

In our modern world, we've been led to believe that the physical, including the body, is the ultimate reality and that external rewards such as material gain and fame are the most important things in life. This focus on the physical has caused many of us to ignore our inner lives. Then, because we are out of touch with our spirit, our days lack meaning and purpose.

Engaging our spirits is a quest that leads us to discover personal harmony, empowerment, and our greatest truth. On this journey we learn to trust our inner guidance that comes from living in tune with our spirits. Engaging our spirit occurs primarily through feeling, so this requires us to be more aware of our feelings than of our thoughts. Once we commit to that awareness, it becomes one of the easiest things we will ever do. It is not so much a matter of thinking or doing as of allowing the truth of who we are to be expressed. The obstacles of thought and resistance will dissolve as we focus on our inner being.

The mind is the doorway, and the body is the manifestation of this process. That is, how we feel is reflective of how we are aligned with the true nature of our spirits. The essence of our being is a space where peace, joy, and love abide. When we feel that joy, are in awe, or experience love, beauty, grace, and appreciation, we are in alignment with our spirits, and our minds and bodies reflect that harmonious engagement as well.

This is why our spirit is the source and foundation of superhealing.

The practice of engaging our spirit allows us the awareness of its qualities throughout our daily lives. It's not necessary to reserve joy and love for a certain day or time; we can experience them continuously. Engagement unfolds uniquely for each of us, whether as the result of an effort to improve our health, reverse a condition, or enhance emotional and spiritual well-being.

Optimal health and well-being is not an end but a process, an adventure along the pathway of self-discovery. I've shared this journey with many people who, even in the midst of deep pain, touched upon their spirits, a part of their being previously unknown to them. Watching this blossoming occur from the turbulent waters of pain and regret has been a privilege for me. We suffer unnecessarily when we ignore our connection to our spirits, to others, to all of life, and to our oneness with the Divine. Opening up to our spirit leads us to a greater knowledge of the positive aspects of ourselves, the truth about our imbalances, an appreciation of our unfolding growth, and an awareness of life's purposefulness and meaning.

This, in turn, enhances our relationships with others and ourselves and affords us a deeper enjoyment of every area of our lives. Aligning with our spirit through being and expression gives us the chance to live beyond the seemingly boring and repetitive nature of our daily existence that has captured a large portion of our awareness. We need to commit to permanent, dynamic change, consistently embracing new perspectives and lifestyle routines, and have the courage to drive our journey in life forward.

It is a challenge to realize that every moment is a gift, that all we truly have is right now, and that living fully present in the moment is the only thing we can ever do. Lingering in the past, dwelling in our minds, and fearing the future interfere with our ability to live in the here and now. The past and the future are memories and thoughts, respectively; they are constructs that, if focused on more than the present moment, keep us out of alignment with our true regenerative and health-enhancing capabilities. Now is the only time and here is the only place in which our ability to superheal our lives resides. While there are many ways to engage our spirits, they all require being fully present in this moment. When we are aware of our spirits, we are living in the present moment, the eternal now.

We're going to take a look at the two primary ways of engaging our spirit: being and expressing.

BEING

Being is a state of dwelling in the high-energy qualities of the spirit— love and bliss—as a continuum of mind and emotion. Being can be experienced and explored through activities such as prayer, meditation, creative endeavors, and sharing through giving, generosity, and compassion.

Engaging our spirit allows us to live more simply and fully. As we do so and begin to consciously express our spiritual aspects, or coherent states of being—joy, peace, enthusiasm, creativity, wisdom, compassion, and generosity—our minds and our bodies will physiologically reflect them.

There is an infinite array of possibilities in the process of expressing our spirit's wholeness. It is not a path of extremes but one of awareness and balance. Engaging our spirit leads us to the peace, fulfillment, and purpose that are our essence. And it will harmonize the seemingly fragmented aspects of our being, shedding light on the wholeness that resides inside. The greatest journey we will ever take is the one we take within.

Life is good. It is a precious gift, and when we begin to consciously engage our spirits, the aspects of being become more frequently present and apparent in our feelings. It becomes apparent to us on a deeper level that the being comes first and expresses itself through a variety of experiences. It is not the situation that brings us joy, but the expression and engagement of our spirit that does so.

I say this without knowing your personal circumstances, blessings, or challenges, because it is all good. It just depends on your perspective. Whatever you are currently experiencing has brought you to the place of desiring and actively seeking more. Otherwise, you would not be reading this book. A good life is not a matter of having no problems. It is about making the challenges softer, and when they come, resolving them with ease and appreciating them more.

Engaging our bodies, minds, and spirits is an evolving process; it changes from moment to moment and is unique to each of us. Superhealing is unique, and its unfolding occurs at the right time for each of us.

EXPRESSING YOUR SPIRIT

You express your spirit when you involve your body and your mind in your own form of being and engaging. This can occur, for example, when you volunteer or when you are creative through writing, singing, dancing, painting, hobbies, and so forth. Techniques for expressing our spirit have been used around the world since the beginning of time. Many of these ancient methods are now employed by medical professionals and have been shown to significantly benefit the healing process of patients experiencing a variety of diseases.

Gratitude

When we are grateful, we are consciously engaging with our spirit. Being grateful heightens our awareness of the blessings we've been given. There is much more to be thankful for than we are usually aware of as our attention is directed to the demands of our daily lives. If you went one by one through all the functions, cells, and biochemical activities of your body, it would take a lifetime to give thanks for them.

Giving thanks, appreciating what we have on a daily basis, can transform our emotional state and provide other powerful health-giving benefits by altering, strengthening, and uplifting our entire physiology.

Thank you is one of the most wonderful expressions we can say and hear. Conveying appreciation is beneficial to us as individuals and strengthens the bonds within relationships.[1] Gratitude is an expression of love rather than judgment. In addition to gratitude, the perspective that all things work together for good, even when the good is not apparent, is a great asset.

I can't give thanks and praise enough to the Divine for all the blessings that have been bestowed upon me. Yet I don't recall all of them, and I suspect that neither can you.

Creativity

We are creative by our very nature. Our creativity is a direct line of expression of the Divine, since all things are created by the all-loving force of which we are a part. I recently heard someone say that creativity is no different from prayer; it is communication with the creator. Every part of our lives reflects our creativity, yet we often remain unaware of its expression. Consciously engaging in self-expression through the arts, music, dancing, writing, singing, and any purposeful activity arouses our natural feelings of passion.

A variety of approaches, from art to music to dance, are now used in clinical settings. Beyond promoting general health and happiness, these activities invigorate the renewal of the mind, emotions, and body. Creativity relieves us of stress in a most wonderful way. Studies say that the stress of work is consuming many of us. Stress can lead to weight gain, elevated glucose levels, upper-respiratory infections, and cardiovascular disease.

I express my own creativity in many ways through my work as a physician. What I do is based not on rote memorization but on a creative engagement with my patient, my inner guidance, my knowledge of medicine, and my holistic superhealing approach.

Nevertheless, ever since I was a little girl, I have wanted to draw and paint. It was a burning desire that remained at the forefront of my mind for decades. During medical school, I learned calligraphy as an artistic expression, because I believed I couldn't draw. A few years ago, I decided to start painting abstract works to appease my desire to create, since I was unable to sketch the beautiful flowers that I wanted to paint. After several months, I became very bored with that particular form of expression. And my desire to draw heightened. Suddenly, the thought dawned on me that if I stopped *saying* I couldn't draw, then somehow I would be able to do so. My mind's perception of my ability shifted in an instant, and I understood how to draw! It was so simple yet equally profound. For years, I'd attempted to draw what I thought the object was—that is, from my logical side—rather than drawing what I saw.

That day, I drew a picture of a beautiful Bengal tiger. I was amazed. And, as they say, the rest is history. Without taking formal lessons, I learned to draw and paint the vibrantly beautiful flowers that I love to behold. I watched a few PBS painting programs and some how-to-paint DVDs, but for the most part, my inner guidance showed me how to express my creativity.

I've hung a few of my abstract paintings next to my floral ones to remind myself of how far I've come and what is possible. My creativity has uplifted me, soothed me, and given me the most rewarding sense of well-being and accomplishment.

Express yourself creatively in whatever way you deem appropriate. Explore new avenues of expression.

Prayer

Prayer is the primary and traditional way all humans communicate with the Divine. Although its true value has been questioned, most people clearly understand its power. A recent survey found that more than 43 percent of Americans pray for their own health.[2]

One of the first studies on prayer that I became aware of was conducted at the University of California at San Francisco Medical School. Dr. Randy Byrd divided 393 seriously ill intensive-care-unit patients, all experiencing various types of diseases affecting the heart, into two groups. The people in the groups were matched for age, type of disease, and the severity of their conditions. Dr. Byrd then asked people from different religious traditions—Catholics, Protestants, and Jews—to pray for the people in one group several times each day. They received only the patients' first names and diagnoses, then prayed for their rapid recovery and the prevention of complications, holding the belief that the prayer would help them recover. Neither the doctors nor the patients knew who was being prayed for. The study demonstrated remarkable results.

Despite their similarities, only the people in the group that was prayed for experienced fewer serious complications, including cardiac arrests, heart failure, pulmonary edema (fluid in the lungs) and pneumonia. Even more amazing, not one person in the group being prayed for died during the study![3]

In addition to prayer, incorporating your spirit into all the mind engagement techniques I outlined in Chapter 3 will enhance your practice and deepen your spiritual connection. Expressing your spirit this way is a form of turbocharging your mind.

Forgiveness

I've saved the best and hardest way of engaging your spirit for last. According to the *Oxford English Dictionary*, forgiveness is "to grant free pardon and to give up all claim on an account of an offense or [a] debt." While one of the most challenging components of superhealing, it is one of the most powerful.

Forgiveness transforms our emotional pain and our attitude toward the offender, replacing negative emotions with positive attitudes, including compassion and benevolence. It requires a conscious decision to transform negative attitudes toward the wrongdoer into positive ones, setting us free from the desire for retaliation, revenge, and estrangement. It occurs with our awareness that we deserve better and that we must let go of the desire for a past that will not change in order to live a greater, happier present.

To make room for engaging our spirit, we must forgive and release the anger and hostility that cannot occupy the same space in our minds as the love that quietly and powerfully, like an ocean tide, promotes and provokes forgiveness.

Forgiveness affords us the opportunity to move on and release the ties that have bound us to our past. The discordant energy of these old unresolved issues impedes and interferes with our path to wholeness. But forgiveness will ease their sting and eventually set us free of the pain and suffering they once caused us.

Forgiveness is not giving permission for the act. Rather it's the understanding that there is something within us that remains unharmed, unchanged, and untouched by it. Mahatma Gandhi contended, "The weak can never forgive. Forgiveness is an attribute of the strong."[4] It is an exercise of releasing the past pains, wounds, and anguish that facilitate disease. We must also forgive ourselves for our own transgressions. Forgiveness aids the process of ending our internal self-rejection and self-loathing.

How do we begin to forgive? How do we forgive those who have caused us great pain? It isn't easy, but it is imperative. When we open our hearts, the areas that need to be forgiven the most are usually not the wrong doings that first come to mind, but the deeper, hidden transgressions that have lurked in the hidden trenches and recesses of the unconscious mind. Because they are so painful and severe, they tend to surface gradually, when we are ready to weather the emotional storm their memories bring.

ENGAGING YOUR SPIRIT

It's important to realize that you are engaging your spirit every moment and in every way. But there is a difference between being aware of it and being unaware of it. The practice of engaging your spirit is equivalent to the practice of engaging your life. Identifying with those aspects of your life that give you a sense of inner peace, comfort, strength, love, and connection will expand and enhance you in a way that nothing else can. In fact, many things you once deemed important will begin to take on a less significant role in your life.

There is a natural sense of well-being that accompanies the awareness of your spirit, leading to your freedom from the imposed (self- or otherwise) limitations that have encumbered joy, serenity, freedom, and self-fulfillment. It is where the ultimate pursuit of happiness and the search for the meaning of life resolve. Engaging your spirit helps you to realize the truth of who you really are, your very being. It results in being fully alive, so that each conscious moment becomes a dynamic process of unfolding and continuously expanding your spirit.

If you want to improve your spiritual health and well-being, I encourage you to explore the following practices. These are but a sampling of ways to engage your spirit. There are many more. Use only those that appeal to you; there is no right or wrong way. You get to decide. Please remember that you are unique, and so is your path to superhealing, so what works for others may not work for you. Be creative!

SUPERHEALING SPIRIT ENGAGEMENT TECHNIQUE #1: SELF-LOVE

Authentically loving yourself, which is not hard, is the foundation of all superhealing. Focusing on loving *you* requires giving yourself attention, acceptance, and appreciation. How do you currently treat yourself? Do you have an inner voice that is very critical and judgmental? Most of us do, and that's okay. But a key ingredient to loving yourself is shifting your attention to silencing that voice and replacing negative thoughts with kinder, more loving ones.

Superhealing Self-Love Engagement Suggestion

Try doing this simple exercise. Just spend ten to fifteen minutes each day quietly reflecting on yourself. Give yourself your undivided attention. Tune in to your thoughts, emotions, feelings, and bodily sensations and fluctuations with acceptance and then appreciate yourself in this moment. Change your judgment of yourself and let the inner critic go.

To accomplish this, get into a quiet state, either through the meditation practices I outlined in Chapter 3, by focusing on your breath, or through awareness exercises.

SUPERHEALING SPIRIT ENGAGEMENT TECHNIQUE #2: BREATHING

Breath is related to spirit. Breathing is usually an unconscious process but a critical one. One of the easiest ways to live fully in the moment is by focusing on your breathing.

In our society, most people breathe shallowly, engaging just the upper part of their lungs. To breathe more deeply, you employ your diaphragm, the muscle that lies between your chest and your stomach. Diaphragmatic breathing more fully engages the spirit because it is a relaxing form of breathing and sends that message of relaxation to the brain. When you are primarily using the muscles in the lungs, that indicates stress.

Superhealing Breathing Engagement Suggestion

To ascertain how you are currently breathing, place one hand on your abdomen and the other on your chest. Watch the way they move when you inhale and exhale: the movement (or lack of it) of the hand on your abdomen indicates whether you are breathing optimally.

If you are not, you can easily learn to do so. Take a breath and feel the air entering through your nostrils and then expanding your ribs as it enters your lungs. Now slightly push out your abdomen, using your diaphragm muscle to help draw the air deeper into your lungs. When you exhale, suck in your abdomen so your diaphragm will help push the air back out. Continue doing this gently and easily.

Once you have mastered diaphragmatic breathing, spend a few minutes every day, with no distractions, and focus on it until it becomes your normal breathing pattern.

SUPERHEALING SPIRIT ENGAGEMENT TECHNIQUE #3: APPRECIATION

My motto is this: Be grateful—"great filled"—for what you have. Ask yourself the following: What am I grateful for? What and who are meaningful in my life? Then express that appreciation in some way.

Superhealing Appreciation Engagement Suggestion

You can write a letter of gratitude to that significant person, or you can engage in one of the most profound ways to express appreciation, which is through keeping a gratitude journal. Doing that on a regular basis for at least twenty-one days will change your brain function and physiology. Finding things to be grateful for is a key positive emotion that will improve your health and reduce stress.

SUPERHEALING SPIRIT ENGAGEMENT TECHNIQUE #4: BEING

I suspect that I don't need to explain to you how to pray, but I do want to share with you how to expand on prayer and other previously described mind-body techniques by infusing them with your awareness of a variety of spiritual qualities. Dwelling in the awareness of or focusing on spiritual attributes is a particular helpful technique in responding to stress and negative thought patterns.

Superhealing Being Engagement Suggestion

Call into your awareness a spiritual quality that you desire to express more consciously in your life—such as love, peace, joy, wisdom, intelligence, abundance, or enthusiasm—as you gently focus your heart on your inner being. You can do this during prayer or meditation or as an affirmation.

SUPERHEALING SPIRIT ENGAGEMENT TECHNIQUE #5: GIVING

Because of the oneness of all things, reflected physically through our interconnectedness, whenever we give to others we are truly giving to ourselves. Thus the ancient axiom "As you give, so shall you receive." But the interesting fact, which I previously mentioned, is that when you give solely to gain a benefit for yourself, the effect is only temporary. You do not achieve long-term enhancements when your motives are not in alignment with your spirit.

Superhealing Giving Engagement Suggestions

There are many ways to give. Explore new avenues for giving of yourself to others: family, friends, colleagues, coworkers, and strangers. The purest and easiest way is to be fully present with a person when you are together.

Committing random and conscious acts of kindness and volunteering on a regular basis, particularly when engaging in the acts from a place of spiritual awareness, are remarkable ways to experience optimal well-being.

SUPERHEALING SPIRIT ENGAGEMENT #6: EXPRESSION OF YOUR CREATIVITY

In my view, there is no difference between picking up a brush to paint and praying. Consciously engaging your spirit by creating is wonderfully uplifting and enjoyable.

Expressing your creativity is not limited to activities like art; it encompasses all of how you live your life. Expression is the foundation of being. To be is to express, and to express is to be.

Superhealing Creativity Engagement Suggestion

There are many ways to express your creativity: drawing, painting, dancing, singing, writing, knitting, crocheting, listening to music, or gardening. You get to decide.

SUPERHEALING TECHNIQUE #7: FORGIVENESS

Forgiving means the end of resentment, anger, and hostility that was caused by an offense (either real or perceived), a disagreement, or an argument. Born from a conscious decision, it entails letting go of the past and the memories of a painful experience that caused you harm and suffering. A bold choice, it is often viewed as being in conflict with our natural mechanisms of self-preservation.

There are many ways to forgive. The most important step is to make the decision to do so. This is not an easy thing to do for most of us, because we are usually entangled by the energy of painful memories, which makes it difficult to let go.

Superhealing Forgiveness Engagement Suggestion

Focus only briefly on past hurts in order to identify something you did or someone you need to forgive. After you have made the decision to forgive, and you feel comfortable with moving forward, you can do one, a few, or all of these techniques.

Expressing Forgiveness Through Meditation

As you follow the meditation steps outlined in Chapter 3, engage your breathing and focus on the concept of forgiveness from your heart. For a few moments, center your thoughts and feelings on the left side of your sternum, where your heart resides. Once your awareness is fully established in your heart's space, ask your heart to dwell in the presence of forgiveness as you call forth, in your mind's eye, the person you want to forgive.

From your heart's viewpoint, look upon the person with compassion, if you can, and when you're ready, speak your piece, whatever that may be. Allow the person to speak back to you, and listen to or feel whatever his or her presence is bringing forth at that moment.

Then when the time is appropriate for you, forgive and release the person to his or her highest good, and release yourself to your highest good as well.

Spend a few moments in silence, allowing your being to feel the freedom and lightness that this process has given to you.

Then take a deep breath and open your eyes.

Expressing Forgiveness by Writing

Write a letter to the person you wish to forgive. You don't have to mail it. Or if you prefer, you can create a forgiveness journal.

Expressing Forgiveness with Visualization

Visualize your act of forgiveness. Talk to the person, then release him or her in love, letting go of the past.

✳✳✳

The bottom line is this: Ultimately, engaging your spirit allows you to be who you are. Superhealing is the journey and adventure of allowing yourself to express your divine capacity and infinite potential.

SUPERHEALING WORK SHEET:
ENGAGING YOUR SUPERHEALING SPIRIT

- How do you currently engage your spirit?
- Which approaches do you find appealing?
- What are the particular benefits you would like to receive?
- How often are you prepared to consciously engage your spirit throughout your day?

Part Four

YOUR
SUPER HEALING
LIFESTYLE

CHAPTER 10

YOUR FORTY-DAY SUPERHEALING ACTION PLAN

Health is a state of complete harmony
of the body, mind, and spirit.
When one is free from physical disabilities and
mental distractions, the gates of the soul open.

—B. K. S. Iyengar

NOW THAT YOU'VE FAMILIARIZED YOURSELF WITH THE BASICS, IT IS time to begin your superhealing adventure.

I created this book to give you the tools and motivation to engage your body, mind, and spirit in order to enhance your health and well-being. With the accumulated information I have shared with you in the preceding chapters, you now have a springboard to help you to create optimal health and well-being,

For some of you, this book may be your first attempt at a more holistic approach to health. For others, this is one of many attempts. In either case, I believe that what is unique about my approach is the continuous engagement of body, mind, and spirit and the recognition of the role that all three play in your health and well-being.

I know for sure that you can superheal your life, and this action plan will help you to do so. I will share with you the foundation and give you examples, but the rest is up to you. You have the freedom to choose how to do it and create your own specific plan of action to make very real lifestyle shifts so you can experience superhealing within forty days, which is the amount of time it takes to set a new habit in place.

Your forty-day plan includes a complementary interactive multimedia support component. I have constructed supplemental podcasts, e-mails, text messages, and a membership site with a social media component, bulletin boards, and chat rooms for peer support. There is participation and goal reassessment at the completion of each twelve-day cycle, and it includes a section on how to manage resistance and several sample action plans. To access these things you will have to go my website, http://www.drelaine.com/superhealing, where you can register to gain access. Please note that this material is only supplemental; the program is completely outlined in this book. The additional information on my website is there if you feel the need for extra support and encouragement.

The steps you will take during the implementation of the forty-day superhealing action plan are as follows:

- **Step 1** (days 1–3): Start with the self-love exercises. Commit to doing only these for the first three days, then continue them throughout the program.
- **Step 2** (day 4): Decide, intend, focus, and act. Fill out the superhealing health review questionnaire and outline your goals.
- **Step 3** (day 4): Review your superhealing work sheets. Decide on your preferences.
- **Step 4** (day 4): Create your superhealing plan.
- **Step 5** (days 5–40): Execute your superhealing plan.
- **Step 6** (on completion of the forty days): Review and refine your superhealing plan.

STEP 1: ENGAGING IN THE MOMENT
THROUGH SELF-LOVE

Even before you create your individualized plan, we're going to begin with love. I would like to help you establish your framework for designing your plan: expressing self-love. Self-love is the foundation of superhealing. If you don't love yourself, you will not have emotional and psychological well-being because you cannot believe that you deserve it.

Ultimately, self-love means to be who you are, your true spirit self. You will truly be yourself only when your personality and your soul align. So I want to invite you to spend three days loving yourself. That will set the tone and increase your likelihood of success.

The keys to self-love are as follows:

1. Attention
2. Awareness
3. Acceptance

How do you currently treat yourself? Do you have an inner voice that is very critical and judgmental? That's okay. Most of us do. Shifting your attention is a key ingredient of silencing the voice and replacing negative thoughts with kinder, more loving ones. Change your judgment of yourself and let the inner critic go.

Here are a few suggestions for self-love in action:

1. Take a quiet relaxing bath, and make it special. Use candlelight, soothing music, and fragrant incense.
2. Spend an evening or a weekend filled with doing the things you like to do.
3. Treat yourself to a massage, a manicure, a pedicure, or something similar.

STEP 2: DECIDE, INTEND, FOCUS, AND ACT

It is important to make a commitment and to honor that choice. This is part of a process I call DIFA: decide, intend, focus, and act. These actions lay the groundwork for your successful participation and are critical to every portion and aspect of this program. Start by designing your program by filling out the superhealing health review.

SUPERHEALING WORK SHEET: HEALTH REVIEW

1. How is your current state of health?

_____

Mind: _____

_____

[Example: My health is okay, I don't have any major health problems, but I am concerned about developing Alzheimer's because my mother had it.]

Body:_____

_____

[Example: I'm pretty tired by the end of every day.]

Spirit:_____

_____

[Example: I'm not sure about my spirit. I need to pay more attention to it]

2. How would you like to improve your current state of health?

Mind: _____

_____

[Example: I want to use affirmations and practice visualization.]

Body:_____

_____

[Example: I would like to have more energy.]

Spirit:_____

_____

[Example: I want to spend more time walking, biking in nature, and gardening, and I'd like to try volunteering with kids.]

3. What does optimal health and well-being look like?

_____

_____

[Example: I think for me, optimal health is when I get up in the morning feeling great, having had a good night's sleep, looking forward to the day, and knowing that my body is prepared to handle anything that comes my way.]

4. How do you want to change your diet and exercise regimen? List your answers here.

_____

_____

[Example: I want to get rid of all processed foods and to eat more vegetables. I already exercise, so maybe I'll do it three times a week instead of once or twice.]

5. How much time each day are you willing to invest in this program, and at what time of day? I recommend at least thirty to ninety minutes in the morning, in the evening, or at night, whatever works best for you.

_____

_____

[Example: I will commit to spending at least thirty to forty-five minutes every day on the program. I will spend fifteen minutes in the morning and fifteen to thirty minutes in the evening.]

6. Are you willing to commit to making this the beginning of a long-term lifestyle shift?

_____

_____

7. Are there any issues that you recognize are currently interfering with your desire to improve your health?

_____

_____

8. What are you willing to do to make this happen?

_____

_____

[Example: I can achieve it by paying a lot more attention to my diet; spending more time in nature; changing my negative thoughts to more positive ones so I won't stress as much as I often do; and spending more time enjoying my crafts, especially making scrapbooks.]

SUPERHEALING WORK SHEET: GOALS

What you would like to experience at the end of your forty-day superhealing action plan?

Mind: _____

_____

[Example: My mind is free of all the chatter. I have peace of mind and a healthier response to life's challenges.]

Body:_____

_____

[Example: I want my body to have more energy and vitality. I want to feel and look younger. My body will be healthier because I plan to lose fifteen pounds.]

Spirit:_____

[Example: I will be more aware of my divine connection to all of life. I will live in greater appreciation of the gifts of my spirit, gratitude, and appreciation. I will be in the presence of each moment with a greater expression of my creativity more frequently throughout each day.]

***

The following outlines the steps to implement the DIFA process, which is designed to help you to build upon your superhealing capabilities.

Decide to Superheal

When someone is ill, he or she tends to focus on not wanting to be sick rather than on getting well. And that's quite understandable if you're living with a health condition. But there is a crucial difference between focusing on wanting to be rid of your illness and concentrating on health and wanting to superheal. This difference may seem subtle, but it is very important. In fact, deciding you want to heal is the most important thing you can do to improve your health.

If you focus on your health, you are literally activating your cells and organs in a way that will help your body to heal. Your decision to superheal assists your body in ways that modern medicine is finally beginning to acknowledge.

You're probably asking, "How do I make that decision?" I recommend that you take a few moments and take an inventory of your life. Consider what is really important to you and how improving your health will assist you. Stop reading for a while and do that right now.

_____

_____

_____

_____

Intend to Superheal

Now that you've decided you want to superheal and be healthy in your mind and body, it is important that you intend to do so. Our intentions shape our lives. They are the energy tracks that unconsciously and consciously channel our thoughts, feelings, and emotions in the direction of our goals.

Take a few moments and focus on intending to superheal and be healthier. Make a heartfelt commitment to do so—whatever it takes.

A key to your intentions is to fuel them with enthusiasm and passion. Passion gives wings to your desire. It will give you the energy and the fuel to reach your goals, whatever they may be. Our passion reflects the will of life, the will to live.

_____

_____

_____

_____

_____

What if you don't feel particularly passionate right now? That's okay, and there's no reason to beat yourself up. It will come eventually.

Focus Your Thoughts on Your Health

Focusing on your health, on getting well, as often as possible is vital. Your thoughts, feelings, and emotions influence your body's ability to heal and regenerate.

To help with this, I like what self-help coaches call affirmations and psychologists refer to as cognitive-behavioral programming. So in addition to the affirmations I've already shared with you in the book, here are more:

1. I can superheal.
2. I intend to superheal.
3. I am getting well.
4. I am getting well now.
5. I have the ability to superheal.
6. My body was created to heal and superheal.
7. I can superheal faster.
8. I am getting well faster.
9. I am getting well faster now.
10. I intend to improve my health.
11. I intend to get discharged from the hospital faster.
12. I am healthy, happy, and whole.
13. My health is improving more and more, and I am getting well faster than I can imagine.
14. My body is strong and remarkable. It is healing now.
15. I am healing now.
16. I am feeling better and better.
17. I am getting stronger and stronger.
18. I am so happy and grateful for all that is functioning in my body.
19. I am grateful for my body.
20. I love my body.

As I mentioned earlier, even though you may feel silly saying these affirmations, if you focus on them for at least fifteen to thirty minutes a day, you will see a profound shift, and it can even change the cells and organs in your body and help them to superheal faster.

Take Action

It just doesn't make any sense for you to choose to become healthy and then act in an unhealthy manner. As you now know, considerable evidence exists that mind-body interventions, as they are being studied today, have positive effects on psychological functioning and the quality of life, and they may be particularly helpful if you are coping with chronic illness.

However, you must commit to taking action and remain consistent with it during this forty-day action plan and beyond. These simple techniques can have a tremendous effect on your mind, body, and spirit, especially when you engage them with a positive mental attitude.

STEP 3: REVIEW YOUR SUPERHEALING WORK SHEETS

Go back to your work sheets from the preceding chapters and review them. They will act as the foundation of the program you design for yourself.

STEP 4: CREATE YOUR SUPERHEALING PLAN

In terms of the structure, there are many ways you can design your program, depending on your particular goals and preferences. If you're just beginning on your superhealing path, I'd recommend following the one I've created with the divisions of this book: Part One focusing on the body, Part Two focusing on the body and mind, and Part Three focusing on the body, mind, and spirit. If you're already engaging, then you may prefer to focus on your mind, body, and spirit all together throughout the forty-day program.

This is your blueprint to take action, and you get to choose how.

STEP 5: EXECUTE YOUR SUPERHEALING PLAN

- Superhealing mind (days 5–16). My advice is to use as many techniques as possible. Variety is the key, especially for the mind. These techniques will provide that. Please refer to Chapter 3.
- Superhealing mind plus body (days 17–28). The purpose of the mind-body techniques is to relieve your stress and to help you function at a higher level. Please refer to Chapters 4, 5, and 6 on nutrition, exercise, environmental changes, and engaging nature.
- Superhealing mind plus body plus spirit (days 29–40). Add the spiritual techniques found in Chapter 9.

STEP 6: REVIEW AND REFINE YOUR SUPERHEALING PLAN

Welcome to your superhealing lifestyle! You have completed the forty days, and now it's onward and upward. This is the time for you to take a look at what has worked, refine your plan, and decide what to do after the initial forty days in order to make your superhealing-lifestyle shift sustainable. The superhealing engagement overview form that follows will help you get started.

SUPERHEALING WORK SHEET: ENGAGEMENT OVERVIEW

Please review the superhealing work sheets you've completed at the end of each chapter. List the techniques and steps you would like to incorporate into your commitment plan. List as many as you would like to use. Remember, this is your personalized plan. There are no wrong answers.

Mind: _____

_____

[Example: Meditate ten to fifteen minutes a day. Write in my journal every day. Use affirmations to reverse my negative thinking. Laugh ten minutes every day, and watch a comedy movie once a week.]

Body:_____

[Example: Learn yoga. Take walks once or twice a week. Eliminate all processed foods from my diet. Use organic products for my hair and body.

Spirit:_____

[Example: Practice gratitude every day. Engage in my creativity at least once or twice a week. Cultivate forgiveness of myself and others.]

FORTY-DAY SUPERHEALING ACTION PLAN FOR BEGINNERS

This plan has been created for those who are just starting to use these techniques. If you're already engaging in some of them, you might want to create a program involving mind, body, and spirit engagement throughout the entire program. I've included a second planning form for those of you who are more advanced. Although self-love is the focus of the beginning of the program, I urge you to include it as a daily practice throughout the forty days.

Superhealing Daily Action Plan for Beginners			
Day 1 Self-love	**Day 2** Self-love	**Day 3** Self-love	**Day 4** Superhealing work sheet review and plan development
Day 5 Mind engagement	**Day 6** Mind engagement	**Day 7** Mind engagement	**Day 8** Mind engagement
Day 9 Mind engagement	**Day 10** Mind engagement	**Day 11** Mind engagement	**Day 12** Mind engagement
Day 13 Mind engagement	**Day 14** Mind engagement	**Day 15** Mind engagement	**Day 16** Mind engagement
Day 17 Mind engagement, body engagement	**Day 18** Mind engagement, body engagement	**Day 19** Mind engagement, body engagement	**Day 20** Mind engagement, body engagement
Day 21 Mind engagement, body engagement	**Day 22** Mind engagement, body engagement	**Day 23** Mind engagement, body engagement	**Day 24** Mind engagement, body engagement
Day 25 Mind engagement, body engagement	**Day 26** Mind engagement, body engagement	**Day 27** Mind engagement, body engagement	**Day 28** Mind engagement, body engagement
Day 29 Mind, body & spirit engagement	**Day 30** Mind, body & spirit engagement	**Day 31** Mind, body & spirit engagement	**Day 32** Mind, body & spirit engagement
Day 33 Mind, body & spirit engagement	**Day 34** Mind, body & spirit engagement	**Day 35** Mind, body & spirit engagement	**Day 36** Mind, body & spirit engagement
Day 37 Mind, body & spirit engagement	**Day 38** Mind, body & spirit engagement	**Day 39** Mind, body & spirit engagement	**Day 40** Mind, body & spirit engagement

FORTY-DAY ADVANCED
SUPERHEALING DAILY ACTION PLAN

Although self-love is the focus of the beginning of the program, I urge you to include it as a daily practice throughout the forty days.

Advanced Superhealing Daily Action Plan			
Day 1 Self-love	**Day 2** Self-love	**Day 3** Self-love	**Day 4** Superhealing work sheet review and plan development
Day 5 Mind, body & spirit engagement	**Day 6** Mind, body & spirit engagement	**Day 7** Mind, body & spirit engagement	**Day 8** Mind, body & spirit engagement
Day 9 Mind, body & spirit engagement	**Day 10** Mind, body & spirit engagement	**Day 11** Mind, body & spirit engagement	**Day 12** Mind, body & spirit engagement
Day 13 Mind, body & spirit engagement	**Day 14** Mind, body & spirit engagement	**Day 15** Mind, body & spirit engagement	**Day 16** Mind, body & spirit engagement
Day 17 Mind, body & spirit engagement	**Day 18** Mind, body & spirit engagement	**Day 19** Mind, body & spirit engagement	**Day 20** Mind, body & spirit engagement
Day 21 Mind, body & spirit engagement	**Day 22** Mind, body & spirit engagement	**Day 23** Mind, body & spirit engagement	**Day 24** Mind, body & spirit engagement
Day 25 Mind, body & spirit engagement	**Day 26** Mind, body & spirit engagement	**Day 27** Mind, body & spirit engagement	**Day 28** Mind, body & spirit engagement

Advanced Superhealing Daily Action Plan			
Day 29 Mind, body & spirit engagement	**Day 30** Mind, body & spirit engagement	**Day 31** Mind, body & spirit engagement	**Day 32** Mind, body & spirit engagement
Day 33 Mind, body & spirit engagement	**Day 34** Mind, body & spirit engagement	**Day 35** Mind, body & spirit engagement	**Day 36** Mind, body & spirit engagement
Day 37 Mind, body & spirit engagement	**Day 38** Mind, body & spirit engagement	**Day 39** Mind, body & spirit engagement	**Day40** Mind, body & spirit engagement

SUPERHEALING ACTION PLAN
ENGAGEMENT AND REVIEW

Congratulations! You've completed the first forty days of your superhealing action plan. Now let's take a look at what served you best during the program.

For each program component, please write down what you did and whether it worked for you as anticipated.

Mind:_____

Body: _____

Spirit:_____

Please review your superhealing goals and determine what you've achieved.

Mind:_____

Body: _____

Spirit:_____

SUPERHEALING WORK SHEET:
ACTION PLAN REFINEMENT

How do you want to change your program? If everything worked as you anticipated, you can skip this step.

Superhealing goal changes: _____

Mind:_____

Body: _____

Spirit:_____

Superhealing engagement changes:_____

Mind:_____

Body: _____

Spirit:_____

SUPERHEALING DAILY LIFESTYLE PLAN

Congratulations! Now that you've completed your forty-day superhealing action plan, you are well on your way to having firmly established the first part of your ongoing superhealing lifestyle. This is only the beginning; this is a lifestyle that will continue to unfold and meet your specific needs as you want. You can review it on a weekly, monthly, or quarterly basis and refine it to help you continue along the pathway to unfolding optimal health and well-being. Your needs will change as time progresses, and you can adjust your plan accordingly.

SUNDAY

Mind:_____

Body: _____

Spirit:_____

MONDAY

Mind:_____

Body: _____

Spirit: _____

TUESDAY

Mind:_____

Body: _____

Spirit: _____

WEDNESDAY

Mind:_____

Body: _____

Spirit: _____

THURSDAY

Mind:_____

Body: _____

Spirit: _____

FRIDAY

Mind:_____

Body: _____

Spirit: _____

SATURDAY

Mind:_____

Body: _____

Spirit: _____

To keep the momentum, I sometimes make a personal spa day or retreat using these techniques. You may want to consider one of the following:

- A superhealing weekend
- A superhealing day
- A superhealing half day
- A superhealing morning

I will also have superhealing retreats and ongoing online and telephonic coaching programs to support you.

This plan isn't written in stone, by any means, but is intended to assist you in creating the awareness of superhealing that already exists in your mind, body, and spirit. As it grows in your awareness, you will find yourself engaging your superhealing abilities without thought.

Afterword: Let Your Superhealing Light Shine

*It is confidence in our bodies, minds, and spirits that allows us
to keep looking for new adventures, new directions to grow in,
and new lessons to learn—which is what life is all about.*

—*Oprah Winfrey*

It's been quite a grand and glorious exploration! As this book ends, I know it is truly just the beginning of your path to optimal health and well-being. Thank you so much for joining me. I am so very, very grateful to have been given the privilege to share the concepts, information, and experiences with you. I did not plan to write this book, but a few months ago the title descended into my mind, without urging, and I knew in that very moment that writing it was the next unexpected and exciting adventure of my life. We've explored the depths of our being, and you've learned how to fully engage your mind, body, and spirit. My primary intention has been to inspire you with the information, techniques, understanding that will remind you of the power that lies within. I've shared knowledge that I trust will ignite your enthusiasm and passion and will serve as the foundation upon which you create your pathways to experience the optimal health and well-being that you desire and deserve. I hope I have succeeded. I pray that you now have a fuller understanding of the truly magnificent being that you are.

My great joy is sharing with you the tools and techniques that will allow you the opportunity to experience the vibrant and vital life you desire and deserve. This work is my life's passionate calling. Thank you for allowing me the opportunity to share it with you. I hope that reading this book has enriched your understanding and enhanced your awareness of the power that your mind, body, and spirit hold within your being. All three possess certain mysteries, miracles, and magic, which I believe will continue to be revealed in our daily lives and in the science that will accompany our unfolding awareness. Your life will progress in unimaginable and remarkable ways as your conscious engagement of your mind, body, and spirit grows.

It is my hope that as you grow in your understanding of who you truly are and how to truly engage your superhealing power, this will become a part of your awareness that is not only a lifestyle lift but also a way of being. I know you can do it. I have absolute faith in you. Remember to be who you really are. Then the light of your spirit will break through the perceptions that are founded in limited understanding.

You've learned much, and now your challenge is to take only what calls you from this book and use it in your daily life. It will change it in ways you cannot imagine, if you open yourself to that possibility.

Because of an unusual weather pattern, we have had have several very cloudy, cold days with dense fog where I live. While I was driving in my car, the fog slowly lifted, the clouds parted, and rays of sunshine rushed through. It struck me that Mother Nature was expressing to me physically everything that I've shared with you. I saw the fog and clouds as physical representations of fear and anxiety and other emotions that impede the perception of the light of our spirit that dwells within us.

May you walk in the light of superhealing and live a life filled with vibrant health and well-being, joy, laughter, happiness, vitality, and fulfillment.

Love and blessings always.

Recommended Resources

Academy for Guided Imagery
www.acadgi.com

American Board of Integrative Holistic Medicine
www.abihm.org

American Holistic Health Association
www.ahha.org

American Holistic Medical Association
www.holisticmedicine.org

American Society for Nutrition
www.nutrition.org

Association for Applied and Therapeutic Humor
www.aath.org

Benson-Henry Institute for Mind Body Medicine
http://www.massgeneral.org/bhi/

The Center for Mind-Body Medicine
www.cmbm.org

Create Write Now with Mari
http://www.createwritenow.com/personal-journaling-resources/

Dr. Elaine
www.drelaine.com

Dr. Mercola
www.mercola.com

The Earthing Institute
www.earthinginstitute.net

Grassroots Health: A Public Health Promotion Organization
www.grassrootshealth.net

Healthy.net: Healthy People, Healthy Planet
www.healthy.net

How to Get Well Faster
www.howtogetwellfaster.com

Institute for Integrative Nutrition
www.integrativenutrition.com

Mind-Body Medicine Practices in Complementary and Alternative
Medicine
http://report.nih.gov/nihfactsheets/viewfactsheet.aspx?csid=102

National Center for Complementary and Alternative Medicine
(NCCAM)
www.nccam.nih.gov

National Wellness Institute
www.nationalwellness.org

Natural Health Line
www.naturalhealthvillage.com

Natural News
www.naturalnews.com

The New Science of Forgiveness
http://greatergood.berkeley.edu/article/item/the_new_science_of_
forgiveness

Nutrition.gov
www.nutrition.gov

Positive Psychology Center
http://www.ppc.sas.upenn.edu/

Spirituality & Health
www.spiritualityhealth.com

NOTES

Preface

1. David Sobel, "Mind Matters, Money Matters: The Cost-Effectiveness of Mind/Body Medicine," *Journal of the American Medical Association* 284 (2000): 1705

2. http://www.cdc.gov/diabetes/projects/cda2.htm

3. The American Heart Association's website: http://www.heart.org/HEARTORG/GettingHealthy/NutritionCenter/Cholesterol-and-Atherosclerosis-in-Children_UCM_305952_Article.jsp.

4. J. B. O'Connell, M. A. Maggard, J. H. Liu, D. A. Etzioni, E. H. Livingston, and C. Y. Ko, "Rates of colon and rectal cancers are increasing in young adults," *The American Surgeon* 69 (2003): 866–72.

5. K. Bottom, M. O'Leary, J. Sheaffer, M. Phillips, X. O. Shu, and B Arun, "Chapter 9, Breast Cancer" National Cancer Institute SEER AYA Monograph p112. Bleyer A, O'Leary M, Barr R, Ries LAG (eds): Cancer Epidemiology in Older Adolescents and Young Adults 15 to 29 Years of Age, Including SEER Incidence and Survival: 1975–2000. National Cancer Institute, NIH Pub. No. 06-5767. Bethesda, MD 2006. G. Null, C. Dean, M. Feldman, D. Raiso, and D. Smith, "Death by Medicine," *Life Extension*, August 2006), http://www.lef.org/magazine/mag2006/aug2006_report_death_01.htm.

6. D. U. Himmelstein, D. Thorner, E. Warren, and S. Woolhandler, "Medical Bankruptcy in the United States, 2007: Results of a National Study," *The American Journal of Medicine* 122 (2009) 741–746.

Introduction: The Foundation of Superhealing

1. Franz Alexander, *Psychosomatic Medicine: Its Principles and Applications* (New York: Norton, 1950), 102, 122, 133, 146, 165, 171, 201. In 1950, Dr. Alexander identified these seven diseases as psychosomatic, and this is what has been taught ever since.
    By and large, it is still accepted that these are the only ones.

2. K. Kieburtz, "Science and Ethics of Sham Surgery: A Survey of Parkinson's vs Disease Clinical Researchers," *Archives of Neurology* 62 (2005): 1357–60; see also R. L. Albin. "Sham Surgery Controls: Intracerebral Grafting of Fetal Tissue for Parkinson's Disease and Proposed Criteria for Use of Sham Surgery Controls," *Journal of Medical Ethics* 28 (2002): 322–25.

3. A. G. Barnett and A. J. Dobson, "Excess in Cardiovascular Events on Monday Mornings: A Meta-Analysis and Prospective Study," *Journal of Epidemiology and Community Health* 59 (2005): 109–14.

4. K. A. Lawler, J. W. Younger, R. L. Piferi, E. Billington, R. Jobe, K. Edmondson, and W. H. Jones, "A Change of Heart: Cardiovascular Correlates of Forgiveness in Response to Interpersonal Conflict," *Journal of Behavioral Medicine* 26 (2003): 373–93; see also G. Affleck, H. Tennen, S. Croog, and S. Levine, "Causal Attribution, Perceived Benefits, and Morbidity after a Heart Attack: An Eight-Year Study," *Journal of Consulting and Clinical Psychology* 55 (2003): 29–35.

5. H. Cerpa, "The Effects of Clinically Standardized Meditation on Type 2 Diabetics," *Dissertation Abstracts International* 499 (1989): 3432.

6. H. A. Tindle, Y. F. Chang, L. H. Kuller, J. E. Manson, J. G. Robinson, M. C. Rosal, G. J. Siegle, and K. A. Matthews, "Optimism, Cynical Hostility, and Incident Coronary Heart

Disease and Mortality in the Women's Health Initiative,"
Circulation 120 (2009): 656–62.

7. J. Boehm and L. D. Kudansky, "The Heart's Content: The
Association Between Positive Psychological Well-Being and
Cardiovascular Health," *Psychological Bulletin* 138 (2012):
655–91.

8. A. R. Herzog, M. M. Franks, H. R. Markus, and D.
Holmberg, "Activities and Well-Being in Older Age: Effects
of Self-Concept and Educational Attainment," *Psychology
and Aging* 13 (1998): 179–85.

9. J. W. Pennebaker, J. K. Kiecolt-Glaser, and R. Glaser,
"Disclosure of Traumas and Immune Function: Health
Implications for Psychotherapy," *Journal of Consulting and
Clinical Psychology* 56 (1988): 239–45.

10. D. Spiegel, J. Bloom, H. Kraemer, and E. Gottheil, "Effect
of Psychosocial Treatment on Survival of Patients with
Metastatic Breast Cancer," *Lancet* 2 (1989): 888–91.

11. A. B. Newberg, N. Wintering, D. S. Khalsa, H. Roggenkamp,
and M. R. Waldman, "Meditation Effects on Cognitive
Function and Cerebral Blood Flow in Subjects with Memory
Loss: A Preliminary Study," *Journal of Alzheimer's Disease* 20
(2010): 517–26.

12. G. Bernatzky, M. Presch, M. Anderson, and J. Panksepp,
"Emotional Foundations of Music as a Non-Pharmacological
Pain Management Tool in Modern Medicine," *Neuroscience
and Biobehavioral Reviews* 35 (2011): 1989–99; see also
D. Knox, S. Beveridge, L. Mitchell, and R. MacDonald,
"Acoustic Analysis and Mood Classification of Pain-
Relieving Music," *Journal of the Acoustical Society of America*
130 (2011): 1673–82.

13. G. Y. Yen, G. Wang, P. M. Wayne, and R. S. Phillips, "The

Effect of Tai Chi Exercise on Blood Pressure: A Systematic Review," *Preventive Cardiology* 11 (2008): 82–89; and N. R. Okonta, "Does Yoga Therapy Reduce Blood Pressure in Patients with Hypertension? An Integrative Review," *Holistic Nursing Practitioner* 26 (2012): 137–141.

14. Hakim Mohammed Said, *Traditional Greco-Arabic and Modern Western Medicine: Conflict or Symbiosis?* (Karachi, Pakistan: Hamdard Academy, 1975), 2–4, http://www .eurekalert.org/pub_releases/2007-05/uom-eng050907.php.

15. Medical FAQ, http://www.medicalfaq.net/what_was _hippocrates_contributions_/ta-123621.

16. Candace Pert, *Molecules of Emotion* (New York: Scribner, 1997).

17. Ibid.

18. Larry Dossey, *Healing Words: The Power of Prayer and the Practice of Medicine* (New York: HarperCollins, 1993), 84.

19. G. E. Schwartz and L. G. Russek, "Energy Cardiology: A Dynamical Energy Systems Approach for Integrating Conventional and Alternative Medicine," *Advances* 12 (1996): 4–24.

20. Victor Fuchs, *Who Shall Live? Health, Economics, and Social Choice* (Hackensack, NJ: World Scientific, 2011).

21. W. C. Willett, J. P. Koplan, R. Nugent, C. Dusenbury, P. Puska, and T. Gaziano, "Prevention of Chronic Disease by Means of Diet and Lifestyle Changes," in *Disease Control Priorities in Developing Countries*, ed. D. T. Jamison, J. G. Breman, A. R. Measham, et al. (Washington, DC: World Bank, 2006), http://www.ncbi.nlm.nih.gov/books /NBK11795.

22. Donald B. Ardell, *High-Level Wellness* (Berkeley, CA: Ten Speed Press, 1986), 94.

23. John Knowles, "Foreword," in Fuchs, *Who Shall Live?*, http://healthcareasthoughpeoplematter.blogspot.com/2011/11/technomania.html.

24. Marsden Wagner, with Stephanie Gunning, *Creating Your Birth Plan: The Definitive Guide to a Safe and Empowering Birth* (New York: Perigee, 2006), 191.

25. Office of Technology Assessment, *Strategies for Medical Technology Assessment* (Washington, DC: U.S. Government Printing Office, 1982), 42.

26. D. Jones, "How Much CABG Is Good for Us?", *Lancet* 380 (2012): 557–58.

27. T. A. Preston, "Marketing an Operation: Coronary Artery Bypass Surgery," *Journal of Holistic Medicine* 7 (1985): 8–15.

28. Dean Ornish, *Dr. Dean Ornish's Program for Reversing Heart Disease: The Only System Scientifically Proven to Reverse Heart Disease Without Drugs or Surgery* (New York: Ballantine Books, 1990), xix.

29. G. Null, C. Dean, M. Feldman, D. Raiso, and D. Smith, "Death by Medicine," *Life Extension* (August 2006), http://www.lef.org/magazine/mag2006/aug2006_report_death_01.htm.

30. Ibid.

31. House Subcommittee, *Cost and Quality of Health Care: Unnecessary Surgery*, (Washington, DC: U.S. Government Printing Office, 1976); see also Agency for Healthcare Research and Quality, "Healthcare Cost and Utilization Project," http://www.ahrq.gov/data/hcup; A. L. Siu, F. A. Sonnenberg, W. G. Manning, G. A. Goldberg, E. S. Bloomfield, J. P. Newhouse, and R. H. Brook, "Inappropriate

Use of Hospitals in a Randomized Trial of Health Insurance Plans," *New England Journal of Medicine* 315 (1986): 1259–66; and A. L. Siu, W. G Manning, and B. Benjamin, "Patient, Provider, and Hospital Characteristics Associated with Inappropriate Hospitalization," *American Journal of Public Health* 80 (1990): 1253–56.

32. Null et al., "Death by Medicine."

33. D. W. Bates, D. J. Cullen, N. Laird, et al., "Incidence of Adverse Drug Events and Potential Adverse Drug Events: Implications for Prevention," *Journal of the American Medical Association* 274 (1995): 29–34.

34. D. U. Himmelstein, D. Thorne, E. Warren, and S. Woolhandler, "Medical Bankruptcy in the United States, 2007: Results of a National Study," *American Journal of Medicine* 122 (2009): 741–46.

35. Centers for Disease Control, "Deaths and Mortality, 2009," http://www.cdc.gov/nchs/fastats/deaths.htm.

36. Nancy Hellmich, "Baby Boomers by the Numbers: Census Reveals Trends," *USA Today* (March 2010); and B. L. Plassman, K. M. Langa, G. G. Fisher, S. G. Heeringa, et al., "Prevalence of Dementia in the United States: The Aging, Demographics, and Memory Study," *Neuroepidemiology* 29, nos. 1–2 (2007): 125–32.

37. Ardis Dee Hoven, "Coping with Baby Boomers, and Staggering Statistics," Amednews (September 2010), http://www.amednews.com/article/20100920/opinion/309209958/5.

38. Ernest L. Rossi and David B. Cheek, *Mind-Body Therapy: Methods of Ideodynamic Healing in Hypnosis.* (New York: W.W. Norton, 1994), 218.

39. Mohandas K. Gandhi, *All Men Are Brothers: Life and*

Thoughts of Mahatma Gandhi as Told in His Own Words
(New York: United Nations Education, Scientific, and
Cultural Organization, 1958), 93.

Chapter 1: Your Superhealing Mind-Body Connection

1. Hans Selye, "A Syndrome Produced by Diverse Nocuous
   Agents," *Nature* 138 (1936): 32.

2. J. M. Koolhaas, A. Barolomucci, B. Buwalda, S. F. de Boer,
   et al., "Stress Revisited: A Critical Evaluation of the Stress
   Concept," *Neuroscience Biobehavior Review* 35 (2011):
   1291–1301.

3. Quoted in Louis Cozolino, *The Neuroscience of
   Psychotherapy: Healing the Social Brain*, 2nd ed.
   (New York: W.W. Norton, 2010), 89.

4. D. Servan-Schreiber, "Somatizing Patients: Practical
   Diagnosis," *American Academy of Family Practice* 2
   (2000): 1073–80.

5. H. H. Klein, "Stress and Myocardial Infarction" [in German],
   Herz 26 (2001): 360–64; see also E. H. Friedman, "Morning
   and Monday: Critical Periods for the Onset of AMI,"
   European Heart Journal 15 (1994): 1727.

6. American Psychological Association, "Stress in America,
   2009," press release, http://www.apa.org/news/press/releases
   /stress-exec-summary.pdf.

7. Lee Iacocca. http://www.brainyquote.com/quotes/quotes/l
   /leeiacocca120043.html

8. Craig Lambert, "The Talent for Aging Well," *Harvard*
   (March-April 2001), http://harvardmagazine.com/2001/03
   /the-talent-for-aging-wel-html.

9. C. Bedell-Thomas and K. R. Duszynski, "Are Words of the
   Rorschach Predictors of Disease and Death? The Case of
   Whirling," *Psychosomatic Medicine* 47 (1985): 201–18.

10. Ibid.

11. Ibid.

12. M. Friedman and R. Rosenman, "Association of Specific Overt Behaviour Pattern With Blood and Cardiovascular Findings," *Journal of the American Medical Association* 169 (1959): 1286–1296.

13. T. M. Dembroski, J. M. MacDougall, P. T. Costa Jr., and G. A. Grandits, "Components of Hostility as Predictors of Sudden Death and Myocardial Infarction in the Multiple Risk Factor Intervention Trial," *Psychosomatic Medicine* 51 (1989): 514–22.

14. N. Geipert, "Don't Be Mad: More Research Links Hostility to Coronary Risk," *Monitor on Psychology* (January 2007), http://www.apa.org/monitor/jan07/mad.html.

15. E. C. Bruce and D. L. Musselman, "Depression, Alterations in Platelet Function, and Ischemic Heart Disease," *Psychosomatic Medicine* 67, supplement 1 (May 2005): S34–S36.

16. S. J. Bunker, A. M. Tonkin, D. M. Colquhoun, M. D. Esler, et al., "Stress and Coronary Heart Disease: Psychosocial Risk Factors," *Medical Journal of Australia* 178 (2003): 272–76.

17. Elida Evans, *A Psychological Study of Cancer* (New York: Dodd, Mead, 1926), http://www.meds.com/archive /mol-cancer/1999/10/msg00897.html.

18. Lawrence LeShan, *Cancer as a Turning Point* (New York: Plume, 1994), 267.

19. Lydia Temoshok, "Personality, Coping Style, Emotion, and Cancer: Towards an Integrative Model," *Cancer Survivorship* 6 (1987): 545–67.

20. Lydia Temoshok and Henry Dreher, *The Type C Connection:*

The Behavior Links to Cancer and Your Health (New York: Plume, 1993), 25, 124–35.

21. Ibid., 5, 155.

22. Ibid., 255.

23. Ibid., 163.

24. Ellen Langer, *Counterclockwise: Mindful Health and the Power of Possibility* (New York: Ballantine Books, 2009), 164.

25. Kathyrn Bold, "Stressing the Positive," University of California Communication (November 2010), http://www.uci.edu/features/2010/11/feature_maddi_101108.php.

26. S. R. Maddi, "Hardiness Training at Illinois Bell Telephone," in *Health Promotion Evaluation*, ed. J. P. Opatz (Stevens Point, WI: National Wellness Institute, 1987), 101–115.

27. Ibid.

28. S. R. Maddi, "The Role of Hardiness and Religiosity in Depression and Anger," *International Journal of Existential Psychology and Psychotherapy* 1 (2004): 38–49.

29. Paul T. Bartone, "Resilience under Military Operational Stress: Can Leaders Influence Hardiness?", *Military Psychology* 18, supplement (2006): S132, http://healthcareasthoughpeoplematter.blogspot.com /2011/11/technomania.html

Chapter 2: Superhealing Mind-Body Research Breakthroughs

1. Ernest L. Rossi and David B. Cheek, *Mind-Body Therapy: Methods of Ideodynamic Healing in Hypnosis* (New York: W.W. Norton, 1994), 218.

2. Candace Pert, "The Material Basis of Emotions: The Binding Tie Between Body and Mind Is a Dialogue of Opiate Receptors," *Whole Earth Review* (Summer 19880, http://www.nancho.net/earthour/bodymind.html.

3. Candace Pert, *Molecules of Emotion:* 72.

4. Ibid., 179.

5. Bruce Lipton, *The Biology of Belief* (Carlsbad, CA: Hay House, 2008), 39.

6. Ibid., 30.

7. Ibid., 32.

8. Ibid., 50, 54.

9. E. E. Espel, E. H. Blackburn, J. Lin, et al., "Accelerated Telomere Shortening In Response to Life Stress," *Proceedings of the National Academy of Science USA* 101 (2004): 17312–15.

10. Ibid.

11. E. H. Blackburn and E. S. Epel, "Too Toxic to Ignore," *Nature* 490 (2012): 1690–92.

12. Ibid.

13. (Damjanovic et al.; Simon et al.; O'Donovan et al. 2009); Valdes et al.; Yaffe et al.; Honig et al.; Panossian et al.; Kananen et al.; Tyrka et al.; Epel.; and Parks, (31) The full citations were initially provided in the manuscript. Here they are again: Several studies involving people ranging from 27 to 65 years with mood disorders, increased stress, poor self-rated mental health, childhood trauma, cognitive impairment and decline, found shorter telomere length when compared to other men. Note: (caregiver stress) A. K. Damjanovic, Y. Yang, R Glaser, etal. "Accelerated telomere erosion is associated with a declining immune function of caregivers of Alzheimer's disease patients," *Journal of Immunology* 15 (2007): pp. 4249–54; (dispositional pessimism) A. O'Donovan, J. Lin, J. Tillie, et.al. "Pessimism correlates with leukocyte telomere shortness and elevated interleukin-6 in post-menopausal women." *Brain, Behavior,*

and Immunity 23 (2009): pp. 446–9; (cognitive impairment and decline) A. M. Valdes, I. J. Deary, J. Gardener, et al. "Leukocyte telomere length is associated with cognitive performance in healthy women," *Neurobiology of Aging*, 3 (2010): pp. 986–92. (Alzheimer's disease) L. S. Honig, M. S. Kang, N. Schupf, et al. "Association of shorter leukocyte telomere repeat length with dementia and mortality," *Archives of Neurology* 69 (2012): pp. 1332–9; (childhood trauma) L. Kananen, I. Surakka, S. Pirkola, et al. "Childhood Adversities Are Associated with Shorter Telomere Length at Adult Age both in Individuals with an Anxiety Disorder and Controls," *PLoS ONE* 5 (2010): e10826. doi:10.1371/journal.pone.0010826; and (psychological stress) E. S. Epel, E. H. Blackburn, J. Lin, et al. "Accelerated telomere shortening in response to life stress," *Proceedings of the National Academy of Sciences USA* 49 (2004): pp. 17312–5.

14. A. O'Donovan, J. Lin, F. S. Dhabhar, O. Wolkowitz, J. M. Tille, E. Blackburn, and E. Epel et al., "Pessimism Correlates with Leukocyte Telomere Shortness and Elevated Interleukin-6 in Post-Menopausal Women," *Brain, Behavior and Immunity* 23 (2009): 446–49.

15. N. Leidy, "A Physiological Analysis of Stress and Chronic Illness," *Journal of Advanced Nursing* 14 (1989): 868–76.

16. C. M. Aldwin, N. T. Molitor, A. Spiro, et al., "Do Stress Trajectories Predict Mortality in Older Men? Longitudinal Findings from the VA Normative Aging Study," *Journal of Aging* 2011, n.d., n.p.

T. B. Herbert and S. Cohen, "Stress and Immunity in Humans: A Meta-Analytic Review," *Psychosomatic Medicine* 55 (1993): 364–79; and E. P. Zorrilla, L. Luborsky, J. R. McKay, et al., "The Relationship of Depression and Stressors to Immunological

Assays: A Meta-Analytic Review," *Brain Behavior and Immunity* 15 (2001): 199–222.

17. J. K. Kiecolt-Glaser, L. McGuire, T. Robles, et al. "Psychoneuroimmunology and Psychosomatic Medicine: Back to the Future," *Psychosomatic Medicine* 64 (2002): 15–28 and J. K. Kiecolt-Glaser, L. McGuire, T. Robles, et al., "Emotions, Morbidity, and Mortality: New Perspectives from Psychoneuroimmunology, " *Annual Review of Psychology* 53 (2002): 83–107. Kiecolt-Glaser, L. McGuire, T. Robles T, and R. Glaser, "Psychoneuroimmunology: Psychological Influences on Immune Function and Health," *Journal of Consulting and Clinical Psychology* 70 (2002): 537–547.K. Kiecolt-Glaser, L. McGuire, T. Robles, and R. Glaser. Emotions.

18. E. R. De Kloet, M. Joels, and F. Holsboer, "Stress and the Brain: From Adaptation to Disease," *Nature Reviews Neuroscience* 6 (2005): 463–75.

19. B. S. McEwen, "Stressed or Stressed Out: What Is the Difference?" *Journal of Psychiatry and Neuroscience* 30 (2005): 315–18.

20. K. Mizoguchi, M. Yurzurihara, A. Ishige, et al., "Chronic Stress Induces Impairment of Spatial Working Memory Because of Prefrontal Dopaminergic Dysfunction," *Journal of Neuroscience* 20 (2000): 1568–74.

21. N. Sousa, O. F. Almeida, F. Holsboer, et al., "Maintenance of Hippocampal Cell Numbers in Young and Aged Rats Submitted to Chronic Unpredictable Stress: Comparison with the Effects of Corticosterone Treatment," *Stress* 2 (1998): 237–49.

22. Ibid.

23. D. Cicchetti and J. Curtis, *The Developing Brain and Neural*

Plasticity: Implications for Normality, Psychopatholgy, and Resilience (New York: John Wiley & Sons, 2006): 21–64.

24. P. S. Eriksson, E. Perfilieva, T. Björk-Eriksson, et al., "Neurogenesis in the Adult Human Hippocampus," *National Medicine* 4 (1998): 1313–17.

25. A. M. Pascual-Leone, A. Amedi, F. Fregni, et al., "The Plastic Human Brain Cortex," *Annual Review of Neuroscience* 28 (2005): 377–401.

26. Ibid.

27. Freedman, "The Triumph of New Age Medicine."

28. J. V. Moseley, K. O'Malley, N. J. Petersen, et al., "A Controlled Trial of Arthroscopic Surgery for Osteoarthritis of the Knee," *New England Journal of Medicine* 347 (2002): 81–88.

29. D. F. Kallmes, B. A. Comstock, P. J. Heagerty, et al., "A Randomized Trial of Vertebroplasty for Osteoporotic Spinal Fractures," *New England Journal of Medicine* 361 (2009): 569–79.

30. C. McRae, E. Cherin, T. G. Yamazaki, et al., "Effects of Perceived Treatment on Quality of Life and Medical Outcomes in a Double-Blind Placebo Surgery Trial," *Archives of General Psychiatry* 61 (2004): 412–20.
    C. R. Freed, R. E. Breeze, P. E. Greene, et al., "Double-Blind Placebo-Controlled Human Fetal Cell Transplants in Advanced Parkinson's Disease" (abstract), *Society of Neuroscience* 1 (1999): 212;

31. C. R. Freed, R. E. Breeze, W. Y. Tsai, et al., "Double-Blind Controlled Trial of Human Embryonic Dopaminergic Tissue Transplants in Advanced Parkinson's Disease: Clinical Outcomes," *Neurology* 52, supplement 2 (1999): A272–A273.

32. German Medical Association, (2010) K. Kuperschmidt, "More Placebo Use Promoted in Germany," *Canadian*

Medical Association Journal 183 (2011): E633–E634.

33.   M. E. Seligman, M. Csikszentmihalyi, "Positive Psychology: An Introduction," *American Psychologist* 55 (2000): 5–14.

34.   B. L. Frederickson and T. Joiner, "Positive Emotions Trigger Upward Spirals Toward Emotional Well-Being," *Psychological Science* 13 (2002): 172–175.

35.   H. Ursin and H. R. Eriksen, "The Cognitive Activation Theory of Stress," *Psychoneuroendocrinology* 29 (2004): 567–592

36.   S. Folkman, "The Case for Positive Emotions in the Stress Process," *Anxiety Stress Coping* 21 (2008): 3–14.

       H. A. Tindle, Y. F. Chang, L. H. Kuller, et al, "Optimism, Cynical Hostility, and Incident Coronary Heart Disease and Mortaility In The Women's Health Initiative," *Circulation* 120 (2009): 656–62

37.   E. Diener and M. Y. Chan, "Happy People Live Longer: Subjective Well-Being Contributes To Health and Longevity," *Applied Psychology: Health and Well-Being* 3 (2011): 1–43.

38.   J. T. Moskowitz, "Positive Affect Predicts Lower Risk of AIDS Mortality," *Psychosomatic Medicine* 65 (2003): 620–626.

39.   B. H. Brummett, M. J. Helms, W. G. Dahlstrom, et al., "Prediction of all-cause mortality by the Minnesota Multiphasic Personality Inventory Optimism-Pessimism Scale Scores," *Mayo Clinic Proceedings* 81 (2006): 1541–4, and T. Maruta, R. C. Colligan, M. Malinchoc, et al., "Optimists vs Pessimists: Survival Rate Among Medical Patients Over a 30-Year Period," *Mayo Clinic Proceedings* 75 (2000): 140–43, and E. Giltay, J. M. Geleijnse, F. G. Zitman, et al., "Dispositional Optimism And All-Cause and Cardiovascular Mortality in A Prospective Cohort of Elderly

Dutch Men and Women," *Archives of General Psychiatry* 61 (2004): 1126–35.

Chapter 3: Engaging Your Superhealing Mind

1. James Gordon and Elaine Zablocki, "Center for Mind-Body Medicine Uses Mind-Body Methods to Limit Stress," *Townsend Letter for Doctors and Patients, Pathways to Healing* (December 2005), http://www.townsendletter.com/Dec2005/pathways1205.htm.

2. S. Bode, A. H. He, C. S.Soon, et al., "Tracking the Unconscious Generation of Free Decisions Using Ultra-High Field fMRI," *PLoS ONE* 6 (2011): e21612. doi:10.1371/journal.pone.0021612.

3. Press Release University of Maryland Study Shows Laughter Helps Blood Vessels Function Better: http://www.umm.edu/news/releases/laughter2.htm.

4. Wakeed A, Salameh and William Fry, *Humor and Wellness in Clinical Intervention.* (Praeger 2001 Santa Barbara, CA).

5. Ibid.

6. A. H. Hunt, "Humor as a Nursing Intervention," *Cancer Nursing* 16 (1993) 34–39.

7. Association for Applied and Therapeutic Humor, http://www.aath.org/general-information.

8. Vicki Woods, "It's Tough Being Down to Three Laughs a Day," http://www.telegraph.co.uk/comment/columnists/vickiwoods/8051978/Its-tough-being-down-to-three-laughs-a-day.html.

9. Ibid.

10. http://www.etymonline.com. http://www.etymonline.com/index.php?term=meditation.

11. National Center for Complementary and Alternative Medicine (NCCAM), "Meditation: An Introduction,"

National Institutes of Health, n.d., http://www.nccam.nih.gov.

12. Herbert Benson, "The Relaxation Response: History, Physiologic Bases, and Clinical Usefulness," *Acta Medica Scandanavica* 660 (1982): 231–237.

13. *Benson and Monks,* ABC, 1985.

14. Herbert Benson, "Temperature Changes during the Practice of g Tum-mo Yoga," *Nature* 198 (1982): 402.

15. The Transcendental Meditation® Program, Benefits Of Meditation. http://www.tm.org/benefits-of-meditation.

16. B. K. Hölzel, J. Carmody, M. Vangel, et.al., "Mindfulness Practice Leads To Increases In Regional Brain Gray Matter Density," *Psychiatry Research,* 30 (2011):36–43.

17. P. Sedlmeier, J. Eberth J, M. Schwarz, et al., "The Psychological Effects Of Meditation: A Meta-Analysis" *Psychological Bulletin* 138 (2012): 1139–71.

18. S. D. Wu, and P. C. Lo, "Inward-Attention Meditation Increases Parasympathetic Activity: A Study Based on Heart Rate Variabilitym," *Biomedical Research* 29 (2008): 245–50.

19. Jon Kabat-Zinn, University of Massachusetts Medical School, Center for Mindfulness in Medicine, Health Care and Society: Mindfulness Based Stress Reduction Program website: Stress-Reduction Page http://www.umassmed.edu /Content.aspx?id=41254.

20. S. W. Lazar, C. E. Kerr, R. H. Wasserman, et al, "Meditation Experience is Associated with Increased Cortical Thickness," *Neuroreport* 16 (2005): 1893–97.

21. E. Luders, A. W. Toga, C. N. Lepore, et al, "The Underlying Anatomical Correlates of Long-Term Meditation: Largert Hippocampal And Frontal Volumes of Gray Matter," *Neuroimage* 45 (2009): 672–78.

22. Andrew Newberg, *How God Changes Your Brain* (New York: Ballantine Books, 2009), 8.

23. Ibid.

24. National Center for Complementary and Alternative Medicine, "Meditation."

25. Ibid.

26. Finch in Van Sertima. C. S. Finch, "Science and Symbol in Egyptian Medicine: Commentaries on the Edwin Smith Papyrus," *Journal of African Civilizations* 10 (1989): 325–351.

27. U. C. Schoettle, "Guided Imagery—A Tool in Child Psychotherapy," *American Journal of Psychotherapy* 34 (1980): 220–227.

28. Carl Jung, Gerald Epstein: Waking Dream vs Lucid Dream, http://drjerryepstein.org/content/waking-dream-vs-lucid-dream.

29. G. Addolorato, C. Ancona, E. Capristo, et al., "State and Trait Anxiety in Women Affected By Allergic And Vasomotor Rhinitis," *Journal of Psychosomatic Research* 46 (1999): 283–9.

30. K. Ahijevych, R. Yerardi, N. Nedilsky, "Descriptive outcomes of the American Lung Association of Ohio Hypnotherapy Smoking Cessation Program," *International Journal of Clinical and Experimental Hypnosis* 48 (2000): 374–87.

31. A. L. Ai, and S. F. Bolling, "The Use of Complementary and Alternative Therapies Among Middle-Aged and Older Cardiac Patients," *American Journal Medical Quality* 17 (2002): 21–27.

32. "Flying," *Aviation, Space and Environmental Medicine* 55 (1984): 196–9.

33. O. Carl Simonton, Stephanie Matthews-Simonton, and James L. Creighton, *Getting Well Again* (New York: J. P. Tarcher, 1978).

34. Alvaro Pascual-Leone and Sharon Begley, "The Brain: How the Brain Rewires Itself," *Time* (January, 2007), http://www.time.com/time/magazine/article/0,9171,1580438,00.html.

35. Ibid.

36. Ibid.

37. M. J. Esplen, P. E.Garfinkel, M. Olmsted, et al., "A Randomized Controlled Trial of Guided Imagery in Bulimia Nervosa," *Psychological* 28 (1998): 1347–57.

T. C. Ewer and D. E. Stewart, "Improvement in Bronchial Hyper-Responsiveness Iin Patients With Moderate Asthma After Treatment with a Hypnotic Technique: A Randomized Controlled Trial," *British Medical Journal* 293 (1986): 1129–32.

L. J. Fick, E. V. Lang, H. L. Logan, et al., "Imagery Content During Nonpharmacologic Analgesia In The Procedure Suite: Where Your Patients Would Rather Be," *Academy of Radiology* 6 (1999): 457–63.

E. Guthrie, F. Creed, D. Dawson, et al., "A Randomised Controlled Trial of Psychotherapy in Patients with Refractory Irritable Bowel Syndrome," *British Journal of Psychiatry,* 163 (1993): 315–21.

H. C. Haanen, H. T. Hoenderdos, L. K. van Romunde, et al., "Controlled Trial of Hypnotherapy in the Treatment of Refractory Fibromyalgia," *Journal of Rheumatology* 18 (1991): 72–5.

J. N. Lyles, T. G. Burish, M. G. Krozely et.al., "Efficacy of Relaxation Training and Guided Imagery in Reducing the Aversiveness of Cancer Chemotherapy," *Journal of Consulting and Clinical Psychology* 50 (1982): 509–524.

R. D. Anbar. *Hypnosis in Pediatrics: Applications At A Pediatric Pulmonary Center.* "*BMC Pediatrics*" 2 (2002): 11.

R. D. Anbar, M. P. Slowthower, "Hypnosis for Treatment of Insomnia In School-Age Children: A Retrospective Chart Review," *BMC Pediatrics* 6 (2006): 23.

M. S. Anderson, "Hypnotizability as a Factor in the Hypnotic Treatment of Obesity," *International Journal of Clinical and Experimental Hypnosis* 33 (1985): 150–59.

A. C. Bakke, M. Z. Purtzer and P. Newton, "The Effect of Hypnotic-Guided Imagery on Psychological Well-Being and Immune Function in Patients with Prior Breast Cancer," *Journal of Psychosomatic Research* (2002): 1131–37.

Chiotakakou-Faliakou, E., Forbes A., MacAulay, S. "Hypnotherapy And Therapeutic Audiotape: Effective In Previously Unsuccessfully Treated Irritable Bowel Syndrome?" *International Journal of Colorectal Disease* 15 (2000): 328–34.

J. Hattan, L. King and P. Griffiths, "The Impact of Foot Massage and Guided Relaxation Following Cardiac Surgery: A Randomized Controlled Trial," *Journal of Advanced Nursing* 37 (2002): 199–207.

Martin Rossman, *Guided Imagery for Self-Healing* (Novato: New World Library, 2000) p. 24.

38. J. Schneider, C. S. Smith, S. Whitcher, "The Relationship of Mental Imagery to White Blood Cell (Neutrophil) Function: Experimental Studies on Normal Subjects," Paper presented at the 36th Annual Convention of the Society for Clinical and Experimental Hypnosis, San Antonio, Texas.

39. J. B. Jemmott, J. Z. Borysenko, M. Borysenko, et al., "Academic Stress, Power Motivation, and Decrease in Salivary Secretory Immunoglobulin A Secretion Rate," *Lancet* (1983): 1400–2.

40. Gerald Epstein, Healing Visualizations: Creating Health

Through Imagery. http://drjerryepstein.org/content/healing-visualizations-creating-health-through-imagery.

41.   Richard Carr and Noah Hass *eds., Art Therapy and Clinical Neurosciences*, 214.

42.   C. Bazzini, A. Ferrari, P. A. Modesti, et al., "Psychological Predictors of the Qntihypertensive Effects of Music-Guided Slow Breathing," *Journal of Hypertention.*, 228 (2010): 1097–1103.

43.   L. Cohen, P. A. Parker, Vence L, "Presurgical Stress Management Improves Postoperative Immune Function in Men with Prostate Cancer Undergoing Radical Prostatectomy," *Psychosomatic Medicine* (2011): 218–25.

44.   S. Cotton, C. M. Luberto, M. S. Yi, "Complementary and Alternative Medicine Behaviors and Beliefs In Urban Adolescents with Asthma," *Journal Of Asthma* 48 (2011): 531–8.

45.   O. Eremin, S. D. Heys, E. Simpson and M. B. Walker, Immuno-Modulatory Effects of Relaxation Training and Guided Imagery in Women With Locally Advanced Breast Cancer Undergoing Multimodality Therapy: A Randomised Controlled Trial," *Breast* 18 (2009): 17–25.

46.   James W. Pennebaker, *Opening Up: The Healing Power of Expressing Emotions* (New York: William Morrow, 1990), 209.

47.   Ibid., 9

48.   J. W. Pennebaker, J. Kiecolt-Glaser and R. J. Glaser, "Disclosure of Traumas and Immune Function: Health Implications for Psychotherapy," *Journal of Consulting Clinical Psychology* 56 (1986): 239–245.

49.   Ibid.

50.   J. W. Pennebaker, and C.K. Chung, (in press). Expressive writing and its links to mental and physical health. In H.

S. Friedman (Ed.), Oxford handbook of health psychology. New York, NY: Oxford University Press, 19. http://homepage.psy.utexas.edu/homepage/faculty/pennebaker/reprints/Pennebaker&Chung_FriedmanChapter.pdf

51. J. W. Pennebaker, J. Kiecolt-Glaser and R. J. Glaser, "Disclosure of Traumas and Immune Function: Health Implications for Psychotherapy," *Journal of Consulting Clinical Psychology* 56 (1986): 239–245.

52. J. M. Smyth, A. A. Stone, A. Hurewitz, "Effects of Writing About Stressful Experiences on Symptom Reduction in Patients with Asthma or Rheumatoid Arthritis: A Randomized Trial," *Journal of The American Medical Association* 281 (1999): 1304–9.

53. Ibid. Claudia Kalb, "Paper, Pen, Power!" (April, 1999), http://www.thedailybeast.com/newsweek/1999/04/25/pen-paper-power.html.

54. David Sobel, "Healing Words: Emotional Expression and Disease Outcome," *Journal of the American Medical Association* 281 (1999): 1328–9

55. Pennebaker, *Opening Up*, New York: William Morrow, 1990; and Kathleen Adams, *The Write Way to Wellness* (Denver, CO: Center for Journal Therapy, 2000).

Chapter 4: Establishing a Superhealing Environment

1. D. Lederbogen, P. Kirsch, L. Haddad, et al., "City Living and Urban Upbringing Affect Neural Social Stress Processing in Humans," *Nature* 474, no. 7352 (June 23, 2011): 498–501.

2. Ibid.

3. National Institute of Environmental Health Sciences, "Lead Poisoning: Is Lead Hiding Here?", *National Institutes of Health*, n.d., http://kids.niehs.nih.gov/explore/pollute/lead.htm.

4. Joel Griffiths and Chris Bryson, "Fluoride, Teeth, and the Atomic Bomb," *Waste Not* 414 (September 1997): http://www.fluoridation.com/atomicbomb.htm.

5. "Mercury Poisoning," *Medicine Net,* n.d., http://www.medicinenet.com/mercury_poisoning/article.htm.

6. National Institutes of Environmental Health Sciences "Bisphenol A (BPA)," *National Institutes of Health,* n.d., http://www.niehs.nih.gov/health/topics/agents /sya-bpa/#a10613.

7. Beth Terry, "Protect Yourself: BPA Is in Metal Cans and Store Receipts," *Blog Her,* (January, 2011), http://www.blogher.com/washing-our-hands-bpa-winter.

8. "Aluminum Toxicity," New York University Langone Medical Center, n.d., http://www.med.nyu.edu/content?ChunkIID=164929.

9. "Eight Household Cleaning Agents to Avoid," *Gaiam Life,* n.d., http://life.gaiam.com/article/8-household-cleaning-agents-avoid.

10. M. Nathaniel Mead, "Benefits of Sunlight: A Bright Spot for Human Health," *Environmental Health Perspectives* 116, no. 4 (April 2008): A160–67.

11. S. L. Hofferth and J. Sandberg, "Changes in American Children's Time, 1981–1997," *Advances in Life Courses Research* 6 (2001): 193–229.

12. V. J. Rideout, U. G. Foehr, and D. F. Roberts, "Generation M2: Media in the Lives of 8- to 18-year-olds," Henry J. Kaiser Family Foundation, (January, 2010), http://www.kff.org/entmedia/mh012010pkg.cfm.

13. S. Kellert and V. Derr, *A National Study of Outdoor Wilderness Experience* (Washington, DC: Island Press, 1998), 4.

14. N. M. Wells and G. W. Evans, "Nearby Nature: A Buffer
     of Life Stress among Rural Children," *Environment and
     Behavior* 35 (2000): 311–30: and N. M. Wells, "At Home
     with Nature: Effects of 'Greenness' on Children's Cognitive
     Functioning," *Environment and Behavior* 32 (2000): 775–95.

15. F. E. Kuo and A. F. Taylor, "A Potential Natural Treatment for
     Attention-Deficit/Hyperactivity Disorder: Evidence from a
     National Study," *American Journal of Public Health* 94 (2004):
     1580–86.

16. N. A. McBrien, I. G. Morgan, and D. O. Mutti, "What's Hot
     in Myopia Research: The Twelfth International Myopia
     Conference, Australia, July 2008," *Optometry and Vision
     Science* 86, no. 1 (January 2009): 2–3.

17. C. Blehm, S. Vishnu, A. Khattak, et al., "Computer Vision
     Syndrome: A Review," *Survey of Ophthalmology* 50, no. 3
     (May 2005): 253–62.

18. "'Five-Minute Memory' Costs Brits £1.6 Billion," Lloyds
     TSB Insurance, n.d., http://www.insurance.lloydstsb.com/
     personal/general/mediacentre/homehazards_pr.asp.

19. Jan Pridgen, "Multitasking: Are We Setting Ourselves Up
     for Failure?" Industrial Extension Service, June 5, 2011,
     http://www.ies.ncsu.edu/news-center/blog/multitasking-are-
     we-setting-ourselves-up-for-failure; and "Infomania Worse
     Than Marijuana," BBC News, (April, 2005), http://news.bbc
     .co.uk/2/hi/uk_news/4471607.stm.

20. National Heart, Lung, and Blood Institute, "2003 National
     Sleep Disorders Research Plan," National Institutes of Health
     (July, 2003), http://www.nhlbi.nih.gov/health/prof/sleep/
     res_plan/sleep-rplan.pdf.

21. National Center for Sleep Disorders Research and National
     Highway Traffic and Safety Administration NCSDR,

"Drowsy Driving and Automobile Crashes," National Highway Traffic, n.d., http://www.nhtsa.gov/people/injury/drowsy_driving1/Drowsy.html#NCSDR/NHTSA; and H. R. Colten and B. M. Altevogt, eds., *Sleep Disorders and Sleep Deprivation: An Unmet Public Health Problem* (Washington, DC: National Academies Press, 2006), http://books.nap.edu/openbook.php?record_id=11617.

22. National Heart, Lung, and Blood Institute, "What Is Sleep Apnea?" National Institutes of Health, n.d., http://www.nhlbi.nih.gov/health/health-topics/topics/sleepapnea.

23. Michael Thorpy, "Sleep Hygiene," National Sleep Foundation, n.d., http://www.sleepfoundation.org/article/ask-the-expert/sleep-hygiene.

24. R. M. Ryan, W. Weinstein, J. Bernstein, et al., "Vitalizing Effects of Being Outdoors and in Nature," *Journal of Environmental Psychology* 30, no. 2 (June 2010): 159.

25. C. Maller, M. Townsend, A. Pryor, et al., "Healthy Nature, Healthy People: 'Contact with Nature' as an Upstream Health Promotion Intervention for Populations," *Health Promotion International* 21 (2006): 45–54.

26. R. S. Ulrich, "View Through a Window May Influence Recovery from Surgery," *Science* 224, no. 4647 (April 27, 1984): 420–21.

27. M. D. Verlarde, G. Fry, and M. Tveit, "Health Effects of Viewing Landscapes: Landscape Types in Environmental Psychology," *Urban Forestry & Urban Greening* 6 (2007): 199–212.

28. R. Hartig, M. Mang, and G. W. Evans, "Restorative Effects of Natural Environment Experiences," *Environment and Behavior* 23, (1991): 3–26.

29. N. Weinstein, A. K. Przybylski, and R. M. Ryan, "Can Nature

Make Us More Caring? Effects of Immersion in Nature on Intrinsic Aspirations and Generosity," *Personality and Social Psychology Bulletin* 35 (October 2009): 1315–29.

30. J. Pretty, J. Peacock, and R. Hine, "Green Exercise: The Health Benefits of Activities in Green Places," *Biologist* 53, (2006): 143–48.

31. John Davis, "Psychological Benefits of Nature Experiences: Research and Theory with Special Reference to Transpersonal Psychology and Spirituality," n.d. http://www.johnvdavis.com/ep/benefits.htm.

32. American Horticultural Therapy Association, (January 2013), http://www.ahta.org/horticultural-therapy

33. Martin Zucker, "Earthing: The Most Important Health Discovery Ever?" *Townsend Letter* (May 2010), http://www.townsendletter.com/May2010/earthing0510.html.

Chapter 5: Superhealing with Movement

1. P. T. Katzmarzyk, T. S. Church, C. L. Craig, et al., "Sitting Time and Mortality from All Causes, Cardiovascular Disease, and Cancer," *Medicine and Science in Sports and Exercise* 41 (May 2009): 998–1005.

2. M. S. Tremblay, R. C. Colley, T. J. Saunders, et al., "Physiological and Health Implications of a Sedentary Lifestyle," *Applied Physiology, Nutrition and Metabolism* 35, no. (December 2010): 725–40; and M. Hamilton, G. Healy, D. Dunstan, et al., "Too Little Exercise and Too Much Sitting: Inactivity Physiology and the Need for New Recommendations on Sedentary Behavior," *Current Cardiovascular Risk Reports* 2 (2008): 292–98.

3. P. A. Gardiner, G. N. Healy, E. G. Eakin, et al., "Associations Between Television Viewing Time and Overall Sitting Time with the Metabolic Syndrome in Older Men and Women:

The Australian Diabetes, Obesity, and Lifestyle Study," *Journal of the American Geriatric Society* 59 (2011): 788–96

4. M. S. Tremblay, R.C. Colley, T. J. Saunders, et al., "Physiological and Health Implications of A Sedentary Lifestyle," *Applied Physiology, Nutrition and Metabolism* 35: 725–40.

5. F. W. Booth and S. J. Lees, "Fundamental Questions about Genes, Inactivity, and Chronic Diseases," *Physiological Genomics* 28, no. 2 (January 2007): 146–57.

6. L. Pruimboom, "Physical Inactivity Is a Disease Synonymous for a Nonpermissive Brain Disorder," *Medical Hypotheses* 77, no. 5 (November 2011): 708–13.

7. Centers for Disease Control and Prevention, "General Physical Activities Defined by Level of Intensity," adapted from U.S. Department of Health and Human Services, *Promoting Physical Activity: A Guide for Community Action* (Champaign, IL: Human Kinetics, 1999), http://www.cdc.gov/nccdphp/dnpa/physical/pdf/PA_Intensity_table_2_1.pdf.

8. J. Woodcock, O. H. Franco, N. Orsini, et al., "Nonvigorous Physical Activity and All-Cause Mortality: Systematic Review and Meta-Analysis of Cohort Studies," *International Journal of Epidemiology* 40, no. 1 (February 2011): 121–138.

9. J. P. Little, A. Safdar, G. P. Wilking, et al., "A Practical Model of Low-Volume High-Intensity Interval Training Induces Mitochondrial Biogenesis in Human Skeletal Muscle: Potential Mechanisms," *Journal of Physiology* 588, no. 6 (March 2010): 1011–22.

10. E. Puterman, J. Lin, E. Blackburn, et al., "The Power of Exercise: Buffering the Effect of Chronic Stress on Telomere Length," *PLoS ONE* 5, no. 5 (May 2010): e10837.

11. C. Werner, T. Fürster, T. Widmann, et al., "Physical Exercise Prevents Cellular Senescence in Circulating Leukocytes and in the Vessel Wall," *Circulation* 120, no. 24 (December 2009): 2438–47.

12. K. I. Erickson, M. W. Voss, and R. S. Prakash, "Exercise Training Increases Size of Hippocampus and Improves Memory," *Proceedings of the National Academy of Sciences* 108, no. (January 2011): 3107–22.

13. L. D. Baker, L. L. Frank, K. Foster-Schubert, et al., "Effects of Aerobic Exercise on Mild Cognitive Impairment: A Controlled Trial," *Archives of Neurology* 67, no. 1 (January 2010): 71–79.

14. Y. E. Geda, R. O. Roberts, D. S. Knopman, et al., "Physical Exercise, Aging, and Mild Cognitive Impairment: A Population-Based Study," *Archives of Neurology* 67, no. 1 (January 2010): 80–86.

15. S. I. Mishra, R. W. Scherer, P. M. Geigle, et al., "Exercise Interventions on Health-Related Quality of Life for Cancer Survivors," *Cochrane Database System Review* (August 2012): 8.

16. S. A. Paluska and T. L. Schwenk, "Physical Activity and Mental Health: Current Concepts," *Sports Medicine* 29, no. 3 (March 2000): 167–80.

17. M. Fiatarone, E. O'Neill, N. Doyle Ryan, et al., "Exercise Training and Nutritional Supplementation for Physical Frailty in Very Elderly People," *New England Journal of Medicine* 330 (1994): 1760–75.

18. A. J. Crum and E. J. Langer, "Mind-Set Matters: Exercise and the Placebo Effect," *Psychological Science* 18, no. 2 (February 2007): 165–71.

19. Ibid.

20. H. Nakata, M. Yoshie, A. Miura, et al., "Characteristics of the Athletes' Brain: Evidence from Neurophysiology and Neuroimaging," *Brain Research Reviews* 62 (2010): 197–211.

21. S. Ungerleider and J. M. Golding, "Mental Practice Among Olympic Athletes," *Perceptual and Motor Skills* 72, no. 3 (June 1991): 1007–17.

22. M. J. Mahoney and M. Avener, "Psychology of the Elite Athlete: An Exploratory Study," *Cognitive Therapy and Research* 1, no. 2 (June 1977): 135–41.

23. D. L. Feltz and D. M. Landers, "The Effects of Mental Practice on Motor Skill Learning and Performance: A Meta-Analysis," *Journal of Sport Psychology* 5 (1983): 25–57.

24. W. E. Mehling, J. Wrubel, J. J. Duabenmier, et al., "Body Awareness: A Phenomenological Inquiry into the Common Ground of Mind-Body Therapies," *Philosophy, Ethics, and Humanities in Medicine* 6, no. (April 2011): 6.

25. E. L. Olivio, "Protection Throughout the Life Span: The Psychoneuroimmunologic Impact of Indo-Tibetan Meditative and Yogic Practices," *Annals of the New York Academy of Sciences* 1172, (August 2009): 163–71.

26. J. K. Kiecolt-Glaser, L. Christian, H. Preston, et al., "Stress, Inflammation, and Yoga Practice," *Psychosomatic Medicine* 72, no. 2 (February 2010): 113–21.

27. Amanda Jekowski, "Yoga May Benefit Patients with Abnormal Heart Rhythm," Cardio Source, April 2, 2011, http://www.cardiosource.org/News-Media/Media-Center/News-Releases/2011/04/Yogamaybenefitpatients.aspx.

28. L. Larkey, R. Jahnke, J. Etnier, et al., "Meditative Movement as a Category of Exercise: Implications for Research," *Journal of Physical Activity and Health* 6, no. 2 (March 2009): 230–38.

29. R. Jahnke, L. Larkey, C. Rogers, et al., "A Comprehensive

Review of Health Benefits of Qigong and Tai Chi," *American Journal of Health Promotion* 24, no. 6 (July/August 2010): e1–e25.

Chapter 6: Superhealing with Nutrition

1. J. T. Cacioppo, L. G. Tassinary, and G. Berntson, *The Handbook of Psychophysiology* (Cambridge, UK: Cambridge University Press, 2007), 211.

2. Ibid.

3. A. Hadhazy, "Think Twice: How the Gut's 'Second Brain' Influences Mood and Well-Being," *Scientific American*, (Febuary 2010), http://www.scientificamerican.com /article.cfm?id=gut-second-brain.

4. D. Y. Kim and M. Camilleri, "Serotonin: A Mediator of the Brain-Gut Connection," *American Journal of Gastroenterology* 95 (2000): 2698–709.

5. "Brain Serotonin Enzyme Finding Might Explain Psychiatric Disorders," *Science Daily*, (July 2004), http://www .sciencedaily.com/releases/2004/07/040709085406.htm.

6. Mayo Clinic, n.d., http://www.mayoclinic.com/health/folate /NS_patient-folate; and Mark Sisson, "10 Quick Tips to Boost Your Serotonin," Mark's Daily Apple, n.d., http:// www.marksdailyapple.com/serotoninboosters /#axzz2H2JdCMFa.

7. L. Van Oudenhove, S. McKie, D. Lassman, et al., "Fatty Acid–Induced Gut-Brain Signaling Attenuates Neural and Behavioral Effects of Sad Emotion In Humans," *Journal of Clinical Investigation* 121 (2011): 3094–99.

8. J. L. Kristeller and R. Q. Wolever, "Mindfulness-Based Eating Awareness Training for Treating Binge Eating Disorder: The Conceptual Foundation," *Eating Disorders* 19 (2011): 49–61.

9. R. D. Berg. "The Indigenous Gastrointestinal Microflora," *Trends in Microbiology* 4 (1996): 430–35.

10. Ibid.

11. Ibid.

12. U. Vyas and N. Ranganathan, "Probiotics, Prebiotics, and Symbiotics: Gut and Beyond," *Gastroenterology Research and Practice 2012* (2012): Article ID 872716, 16 pages, 2012. doi:10.1155/2012/872716; Y. Miyake and K. Yamamoto, "Role of Gut Microbiota in Liver Diseases," *Hepatology Research* 43 (2012): 139–146 ; and A. Orlando and F. Russo, "Intestinal Microbiota, Probiotics and Human Gastrointestinal Cancers," *Journal of Gastrointestinal Cancer* 44 (2012): 121–131.

13. M. Messaoudi, N. Violle, J. F. Bisson, et al., "Beneficial Psychological Effects of a Probiotic Formulation (*Lactobacillus heveticus* R0052 and *Bifidobacterium longum* R0175) in Healthy Human Volunteers," *Gut Microbes* 2 (2011): 254–61.

14. M. Messaoudi, R. Lalonde, and N. Violle, "Assessment of Psychotropic-Like Properties of a Probiotic Formulation (*Lactobacillus helveticus* R0052 and *Bifidobacterium longum* R0175) in Rats and Human Subjects," *British Journal of Nutrition* 105 (2011): 755–64.

15. P. Berick, E. F. Verdu, and J. A. Foster, "Chronic Gastrointestinal Inflammation Induces Anxiety-Like Behavior and Alters Central Nervous System Biochemistry in Mice," *Gastroenterology* 139 (2010): 2102–12.

16. J. Faher, I. Kovacs, and C. B. Gabrieli, "Role of Gastrointestinal Inflammations in the Development and Treatment of Depression," *Orvosi Hetilap* 152 (2011): 1477–85.

17. Max Gerson, The Gerson Therapy author's website, n.d.,
    http://gerson.org/gerpress/the-gerson-therapy/.

18. D. G. Blanchflower, A. J. Oswald, and S. Stewart-
    Brown, "Is Psychological Well-Being Linked to the
    Consumption of Fruit and Vegetables?", *Social Indicators
    Research* (October 2012), http://www.nber.org/papers/
    w18469] http://www.Andrewoswald.com/docs/
    October2FruitAndVeg2012BlanchOswaldStewartBrown.pdf.

19. S. Nair, W. Li, and A. N. Kong, "Natural Dietary Anti-Cancer
    Chemopreventive Compounds: Redox-Mediated Differential
    Signaling Mechanisms in Cytoprotection of Normal Cells
    ersus Cytotoxicity in Tumor Cells," *Acta Pharmacolicga
    Sinica* 28 (2007): 459–72.

20. S. Shankar, D. Kumar, and R. K. Srivastava, "Epigenetic
    Modifications by Dietary Phytochemicals: Implications for
    Personalized Nutrition," *Pharmacology and Therapeutics*
    (November 2012): ii.

21. A. Ascherio, H. Chen, M. G. Weisskopf, et al., "Pesticide
    Exposure and Risk for Parkinson's Disease," *Annals of
    Neurology* 60 (2006): 197–203.

22. Russell Blaylock, *Excitotoxins: The Taste That Kills* (Sante Fe,
    NM: Health Press, 1996), 49.

23. Joseph Mercola, review of *The Whole Soy Story: The Dark
    Side of America's Favorite Health Food*, by Kaayla T. Daniel,
    (July 2008), http://articles.mercola.com/sites/articles/
    archive/2008/07/17/the-whole-soy-story-the-dark-side-of-
    america-s-favorite-health-food.aspx.

24. F. A. Popp, "Properties of Biophotons and Their Theoretical
    Implications," *Indian Journal of Experimental Biology* 5
    (May 2003): 391–402; F. A. Popp, Q. Gu, and K. H. Li,
    "Biophoton Emission: Experimental Background and

Theoretical Approaches," *Modern Physics Letters B* 8, nos. 21–22 (1994): 1269–96; F. A. Popp, "Biophotons— Background, Experimental Results, Theoretical Approach and Applications," *Research Advances in Photochemistry and Photobiology* 1 (2000): 31–41; and S. Cohen and F. A. Popp, "Biophoton Emission of the Human Body," *Journal of Photochemistry and Photobiology B: Biology* 40 (1997): 187–89.

25. Cohen and Popp, "Biophoton Emission of the Human Body," 440.

26. G. L. Bowman, L. C. Silbert, D. Howieson, et al., "Nutrient Biomarker Patterns, Cognitive Function, and MRI Measures of Brain Aging," *Neurology* 78 (2012): 241–49.

27. Mercola, review of *The Whole Soy Story*.

28. D. R. Davis, M. D. Epp, and H. D.Riordan, "Changes in USDA Food Composition Data for 43 Garden Crops, 1950 to 1999," *Journal of the American College of Nutrition* 23 (2004): 669–82.

29. Susan Rinkunas, "Pop This Supplement to Stay Young," *Women's Health*, n.d., http://www.womenshealthmag.com/health/fish-oil-benefits.

30. "Vitamin D Weight Loss Information," Vitamin D Weight Loss, n.d., http://www.vitamindweightloss.net.

31. Mike Adams, "Astaxanthin: The Little-Known Miracle Nutrient for Inflammation, Anti-Aging, Athletic Endurance, and More," *Natural News*, n.d., http://www.naturalnews.com/023177_astaxanthin_antioxidants.html.

32. Jonathan Benson, "Scientists Call Resveratrol a 'Miracle Molecule,'" *Natural News*, (September, 2012), http://www.naturalnews.com/037294_resveratrol_miracle_nutrient.html.

33. New York University Langore Medical Center, "L-Theanine," http://www.med.nyu.edu/content?ChunkIID=653856]

Chapter 7: Your Superhealing Spirit-Body Connection

1. A. K. Bansal, and S. D. Sharma, "Can Spiritual Health Be Quantified: A Simple Idea," paper presented at the International Conference on Statistics, Combinatory, and Related Areas, University of Southern Maine, Portland, October 3–5, 2003.

2. M. N. Shiota, S. L. Neufield, W. H. Yeung, et al., "Feeling Good: Autonomic Nervous System Responding in Five Positive Emotions," *Emotion* 11 (2011): 1368–78.

3. C. Chida and A. Steptoe, "Positive Psychological Well-Being and Mortality: A Quantitative Review of Prospective Observational Studies," *Psychosomatic Medicine* 70, no. (September 2008): 741–56.

4. A. Steptoe, "Psychophysiological Contributions to Behavioral Medicine and Psychosomatics," in *The Handbook of Psychophysiology*, ed. J. T. Cacioppo, L. G. Tassinary, and G. Bernston, 3rd ed., 723–25 (New York: Cambridge University Press, 2007).

5. E. Diener and M. Y. Chan, "Happy People Live Longer: Subjective Well-Being Contributes to Health and Longevity," *Applied Psychology: Health and Well-Being* 3 (2011): 1–43.

6. J. Lacey and B. C. Lacey, "Two-Way Communication Between the Heart and the Brain: Significance of Time Within the Cardiac Cycle," *American Psychologist* (February 1978): 99–113.

7. R. McCraty. "Influence of Cardiac Afferent Input on Heart-Brain Synchronization and Cognitive Performance," *International Journal of Psychophysiology* 45 (2002): 72–73.

8. E. Diener, N. Weiting, J. Harter, et al., "Wealth and

Happiness Across the World: Material Prosperity Predicts
Life Evaluation, Whereas Psychosocial Prosperity Predicts
Positive Feeling," *Journal of Personality and Social Psychology*
99 (2010): 52–61.

Chapter 8: The Superhealing Power of Love and Relationships

1. R. M. Nerem, M. J. Levesque, and J. F. Cornhill, "Social
   Environment as a Factor in Diet-Induced Atherosclerosis,"
   Science 208 (1980): 1475–76.

2. T. Field, "Touch for Socioemotional and Physical Well-
   Being: A Review," *Developmental Review* 30 (2010): 367–83.

3. T. Field, "Massage Therapy Facilitates Weight Gain in
   Preterm Infants," *Current Directions in Psychological
   Science* 10 (2001): 51–54; T. Field, S. M. Schanberg,
   F. Scafidi, C. R. Bauer, N. V. Lahr, R. Garcia, J. Nystrom, and
   C. M. Kuhn, "Tactile/Kinesthetic Stimulation Effects on
   Preterm Neonates," *Pediatrics* 77 (1986): 654–58; T. Field,
   N. Grizzle, F. Scafidi, S. Abrams, S. Richardson, C. Kuhn, and
   S. Schanberg, "Massage Therapy for Infants of Depressed
   Mothers," *Infant Behavior and Development* 19 (1996):
   107–12; M. Hernandez-Reif, T. Field, J. Krasnegor, and
   H. Theakston, "Lower Back Pain Is Reduced and Range of
   Motion Increased After Massage Therapy," *International
   Journal of Neuroscience* 106 (2001): 131–45; M. Hernandez-
   Reif, T. Field, J. Krasnegor, and H. Theakston, "High Blood
   Pressure and Associated Symptoms Were Reduced by
   Massage Therapy," *Journal of Bodywork and Movement
   Therapies* 4 (2000): 31–38; M. Diego and T. Field, "Moderate
   Pressure Massage Elicits a Parasympathetic Nervous System
   Response," *International Journal of Neuroscience* 119 (2009):
   630–39; M. Hernandez-Reif, J. Dieter, T. Field, B. Swerdlow,
   and M. Diego, "Migraine Headaches Are Reduced by
   Massage Therapy," *International Journal of Neuroscience*

96 (1998): 1–11; and G. Ironson, T. M. Field, F. Scafidi, M. Hashimoto, M. Kumar, A. Kumar, A. Price, A. Goncalves, I. Burman, C. Tetenman, R. Patarca, and M. A. Fletcher, "Massage Therapy Is Associated with Enhancement of the Immune System's Cytotoxic Capacity," *International Journal of Neuroscience* 84 (1996): 205–17. These studies can be found at http://www6.miami.edu/touch-research/research.html.

4. M. J. Hertenstein, J. M. Verkamp, , A.M. Kerestes, et al., "The Communicative Functions of Touch in Humans, Nonhuman Primates and Rats: A Review and Synthesis of the Empirical Research," *Genetic, Social, and General Psychology Monographs* 132 (2006): 5–94.

5. T. Field, "American Adolescents Touch Each Other Less and Are More Aggressive Toward Their Peers Compared with French Adolescents," *Adolescence* 34 (1999): 753–58.

6. T. Field, "Preschoolers in America Are Touched Less and Are More Aggressive Than Preschoolers in France," *Early Child Development and Care* 151 (1999): 1–17.

7. J. S. House, K. R. Landis, D. Umerson, "Social Relationships and Health," *Science* 29 (19889): 540–45.

8. W. Woods, N. Rhodes, and M. Whelan, "Sex differences in Positive well-being a Consideration of Emotional Style and Marital Status," *Psychological Bulletin* 106 (1989): 249–264.

9. J. C. Coyne, M. J. Rohrbaugh, V. Shoham, et al., "Prognostic Importance of Marital Quality for Survival of Congestive Heart Failure," *American Journal of Cardiology* 88 (2001): 526–529, and T. F. Robles and J. K Kiecolt-Glaser, "The Physiology of Marriage: Pathways to Health," *Physiology and Behavior* 79 (2003): 409–416.

10. R. W. Bartrop, L, Lazarus, L. Luckhurst, et al., "Depressed

Lymphocyte Function After Bereavement," *Lancet* 8016 (1977): 834–836.

11. U. Goldbourt and J. H. Medalie, et al, " Isolated Low HDL Cholesterol As a Risk Factor for Coronary Heart Disease Mortality," *Arteriosclerosis, Thrombosis and Vascular Biology* 17 (1997): 107–113.

12. House, Landis, and Umberson, Social Relationships and Health, (previously cited)

13. D. Spiegel, J. Bloom, H. Kraemer, et al., "Effect of Psychosocial Treatment on Survival Of Patients With Metastatic Breast Cancer," *The Lancet* 2, (1989). 888–91.

14. B. Egolf, J. Lasker, S. Wolf, et al., "The Roseto Effect: A 50-Year Comparison of Mortality Rates," *American Journal of Public Health* 82 (1992): 1089–92, and D. Ornish, S. E. Brown, J. H. Billings, et al, "Can Lifestyle Changes Reverse Coronary Artery Disease?" *Lancet* 336 (1990): 129–133 and D. Spiegel, J. Bloom, H. Kraemer, et al., "Effect of Psychosocial Treatment on Survival Of Patients With Metastatic Breast Cancer," *The Lancet* 2, (1989): 888–91.

15. C. N. Dewall, G. Macdonald, G. D. Webster, et al., "Acetaminophen Reduces Social Pain: Behavioral and Neural Evidence," *Psychological Science* 21 (2010): 931–37.

16. B. Egolf, J. Lasker, S. Wolf, et al., "The Roseto Effect: A 50-Year Comparison of Mortality Rates," *American Journal of Public Health* 82 (1992): 1089–92.

17. J. A. Coan, H. S. Schaefer, and R. J. Davidson, "Lending a Hand: Social Regulation of the Neural Response to Threat," *Psychological Science* 17, no. 12 (2006): 1032–39.

18. Allan Luks and Peggy Payne, *The Healing Power of Doing Good: The Health and Spiritual Benefits of Helping Others* (Fawcett Columbine: New York, 1991).

19. S. Konrath, A. Fuhrel-Forbis, A. Lou, et al., "Motives for Volunteering Are Associated with Mortality Risk in Older Adults," *Health Psychology* 31 (2012): 87–96.

20. T. Field, M. Hernandez-Reif, O. Quintino, et al., "Elder Retired Volunteers Benefit from Giving Massage Therapy to Infants." *Journal of Applied Gerontology* 17 (1998): 229–39.

21. R. A. Emmons, *Thanks! How the New Science of Gratitude Can Make You Happier* (Boston: Houghton-Mifflin, 2007).

22. Ibid.

Chapter 9: Engaging Your Superhealing Spirit

1. M. Y. Bartlett, P. Condon, J. Cruz, et al., "Gratitude: Prompting Behaviours That Build Relationships," Cognition and Emotion 26 (2012): 2–13; S. B. Algoe, J. Haidt, and S. L Gable, "Beyond Reciprocity: Gratitude and Relationships in Everyday Life," Emotion 8 (2008): 425–29; N. M. Lambert, M. S. Clark, J. Durtschi, et al., "Benefits of Expressing Gratitude: Expressing Gratitude to a Partner Changes One's View of the Relationship," Psychological Science 21 (2010): 573–80; and Emmons, J. E.Wilkinson, R. B. Saper, A. K. Rosenthal, et al., "Prayer For Health And Primary Care: Results From The 2002 National Health Interview Survey," *Family Medicine,* 40 (2008): 638–44.

2. R. C. Byrd, "Positive Therapeutic Effects of Intercessory Prayer in a Coronary Care Unit Population," *Southern Medical Journal* 81 (1988): 826–29.

3. Gandhi, *All Men Are Brothers,* 155.

4. Ibid.

Index

ABOUT THE AUTHOR

ELAINE FERGUSON, MD, IS AN IVY LEAGUE-EDUCATED PHYSICIAN and a graduate of Brown University and the Duke University School of Medicine. She did her residency training at the University of Chicago's Hospitals and Clinics and has practiced holistic medicine for over two decades in the Chicago area both in private practice and as a corporate administrator. Her career highlights include practicing medicine at the Cancer Treatment Centers of America. She was also the founding medical director of one of the nation's first alternative medicine independent practice associations—designed to provide primary care to a major insurance carrier.

In her current position as Senior Medical Director for the U.S. Postal Service Great Lakes Area, which includes Michigan, Indiana, Illinois, Wisconsin, Missouri, and Minnesota, she plays an administrative role in which she's responsible for ensuring the well-being of employees, as well as customers, and she supervises the USPS National Health Promotion Program. Dr. Ferguson also has a consulting practice, One Health, where she she consults with health care companies and other businesses to improve health related outcomes.

For several years, Dr. Ferguson wrote a column, "Spirituality and Health," for *Alternative Medicine Digest Magazine*. She currently writes for her blog at DrElaine.com. She is creator of a line of educational audios and workbooks for people with various physical conditions, such as diabetes, hypertension, post-surgical recovery, called "How to Get Well Faster."

Dr. Ferguson has lectured on holistic medicine at colleges, universities, and medical schools—among them Brown University, Medical College of Ohio, and the University of Chicago—and at international medical conferences. In the early 1990s, she taught mind/

body medicine at DePaul University's Foundations of Holistic Health (now-defunct), one of the first graduate level holistic medicine programs in the United States. She also taught a course on community health at Roosevelt University in Chicago.

Dr. Ferguson testified on a panel of experts at congressional hearings convened by Congressman Louis Stokes of Cleveland to explore advances in nutrition and complementary and alternative medicine (NCAM). She was also a member of the American Cancer Society's, Committee on Alternative Cancer Therapies.

In her spare time, Dr. Ferguson paints, gardens, and engages in the textile arts. She lives with her husband, Victor Johnson, in Valparaiso, Indiana.

To learn more visit her website DrElaine.com.